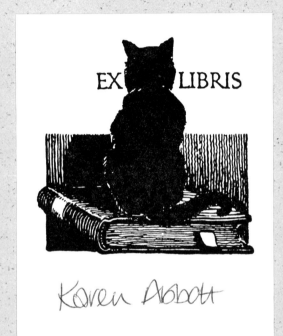

EX LIBRIS

Karen Abbott

Hygieia

a woman's herbal

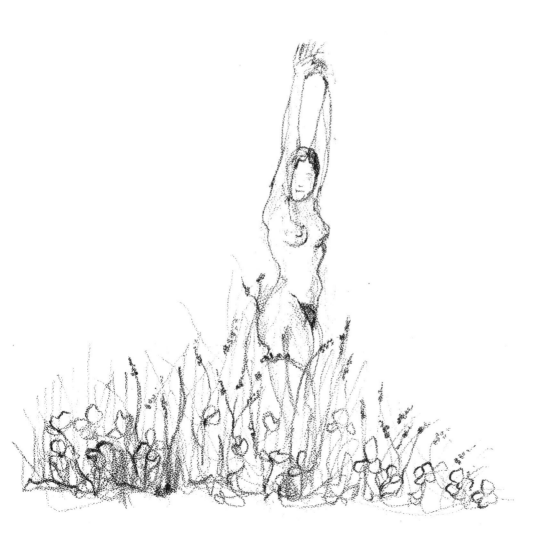

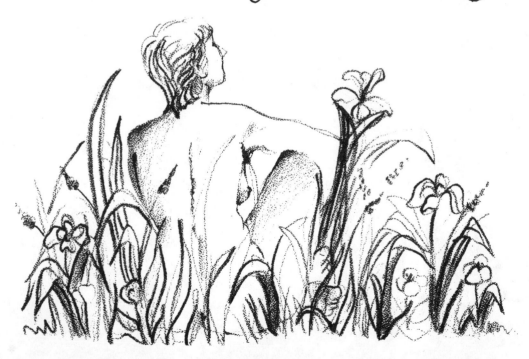

CREDITS

❖ Book Design © Tamara Slayton Glenn

❖ Photographs on pages 5, 12, 140 by Patricia Jolley
　　　　　· pages 114, 118, 210 by Michael Medvin
　　　　　· page 214 by Steven Glenn
　　　　　· page 186 by Jeannine Parvati
　　　　　· page 98 by Michael Markowitz

❖ Drawings ～ on page viii by Loi Medvin
　　　　　· pages 42-48, 56-58, 76-78, 100, 102-109, 111 by Quill Cleaver

❖ Dreams from Nadine Soffer

❖ Typesetting by Georgeanne of Guerneville Graphics,
　　　　and Hinda Kapust

❖ A FREESTONE COLLECTIVE BOOK ❖

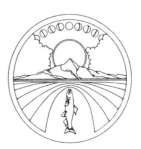

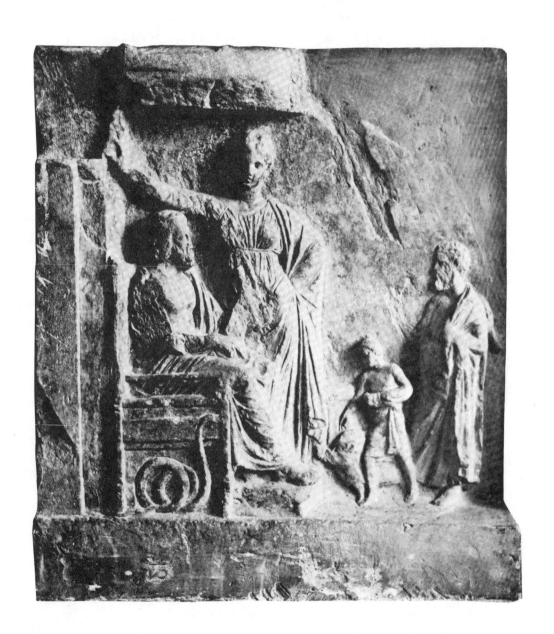

The Feminine and Healing

What I have explored in the process of making this book is the relationship between the feminine and healing. The movement into this domain was heralded by a visitation from Hygieia, the Greek goddess of healing. What is left unsaid in these musings is the rather incestuous nature of Hygieia's work with her father, Aesclepius. The story is an elusive one, an Eleusian one, as far as my readings into myth are concerned. For it appears to be that Hygieia either worked as a healing goddess in conjunction with her father, or with her father and mother. Some writers seem to believe that Hygieia was actually an incarnation of Athena and linked with ancient moon-cults. Others write that she actually assumed her own mother's, Epione's, position in her father's eyes. Nevertheless, the art of the Greeks and Romans often shows Hygieia with her father and mother engaged in healing as a Trimurti, a trinity of healers. Imaginally, I would venture to suggest that from Hygieia's perspective, this trinity of psychic physicians points to the necessity of rooting out the "cause" or geneology of illness. My hunch is that a lot of sickness in the female being is connected with life-force/sexual energy of one's parents. This may hold true for men as well. The relationship of female sexuality and healing is to be the topic of my enquiry in future work. The question presented by James Hillman to me is provocative--and that is, "Just how dirty is Hygieia?"

Basically, what I have come to understand about soul education is the necessity to make available information and to inspire to wisdom all sentient beings. And awaken in each of us our connection with the invisible or subtle body (the imaginal) that is so reflective of personal health. I am struck over and over again in my counselings and sharings with women the essences of their dramas with gynecologists. Through the veils of anger and blame a very important message shows itself. And that is just perhaps, when our sufferings become intolerable (eg. a virulent vaginal infection), we visit the doctor to bring about a healing in not only our bodies but our souls as well. And not only via ritualistic confessions but through active humiliation and shame. This is how I perceive this idea in operation--she has pain in her cunt, she can't help herself, she seeks the expert, he names it, she suffers from his lack of caring, she sees the mask of dis-ease reflected back upon her soul--and then it's not just her cunt that is in pain, but the realization comes that it is her soul that is hurting too. So my theory is that women patronize insensitive male gynecologists to bring about this union between the imaginal and the physical bodies, and it is a wedding of the most curious sort.

Visiting a gynecologist is by nature a sexual experience with all the inherent possibilities our genitals symbolize. And the passion is best expressed by traditional gynecological practices such as cutting and burning of the female sexual organs. "Passion shows us the seamy side of things. It shows us the imprint of cutting and healing." B. Jager (from "The Phenomenolgy of Passion").

With Hygieia as an image alive with whom we relate during the healing process, there is the possibility of becoming one's own mother. The original imprint of cutting and healing is the severance from the mother via umbilical cord. The connection with power, the third chakra, the lower boiler, and our ability to move about in the world as an individual is implicated here. As is our sense of grounding through shame, helplessness and other Mother-related dependencies. The implications of this excite me no end. The place for the health advocate is **within this context.**   From one perspective, it is the mystery of the Eleusians--that the secret of immortality is expressed in the image of woman giving birth to herself, the merging of the daughter and the mother. E. Esther Harding's statement of what is a virgin is relevent here also. She described her as "woman complete unto herself." There is a quality of virginal purity in women healing themselves, in my experience. And a quality of greatest compassion. With tenderly caring for one's own growing or evolving psychic-physical world, as every mother of young children knows, there comes the development of greater and deeper qualities of human-ness. We who are learning how to heal ourselves are also learning how to value all of life's experiences and our infinite capability to be responsive to (responsible for) whatever dilemma our souls may lead us.

So I see this creative project, the book Hygieia: A WOMAN'S HERBAL, as an attempt to translate from the soul's point of view the phenomenom of holistic health as it relates to women, and many aspects of the feminine. The book was written for the mythical "everywoman"--in my fantasy she is a sometimes fertile, creative being and rarely a victim. That is why the idea of what could be seen solely as horrendous medical practices upon defenseless women patients needs re-visioning. For as great a motivator as anger and blame may be, it does mask the value of seeing our humiliations at the hands of gynecologists (or obstetricians) as important expressions and experiences of our soul. I know that I personally could not heal myself or evoke this ability in any of my sisters when my energy was psychically reacting against the patriarchy. For the underlying metaphor of healing is union. I took the Delphic oracle's words to Apollo seriously--The Wounder Heals--and by understanding my part in the medical drama, I was able to let go my grievances with the patriarchal style of healing. Up til then, all the knowledge I'd gathered about the workings of the body and health remained tied-up as information. When I could temper this study with the knowings of my soul, and allow the mind-stuff to be touched by my heart, the "wicca" or wise woman healer was evoked. And my wise woman would accept imaginally the father as healer and understand that he, too, is doing the best that he can. As are we all.

HYGIEIA SAYS:
"THE WOUND
REVEALS
THE CURE."

Special Thanks to the herbal ladies who inspired me into this gentle art of healing ~ Juliette de Baircli Levy ~ Jeanne Rose ~ Lilyan Garcia McClure ~ Rosemary Gladstar ~ Nan Koehler ~ Rita Weinstein ~ Maxine Jarrel ~ Rob Menzonne ~ and our three daughters ~ Shobha, Prabha, Abha, who share the world of ideas & flower fairies with me. ~ And a very full appreciation for Vishnu Dass, the One I love, who opens my being to the Divine every day

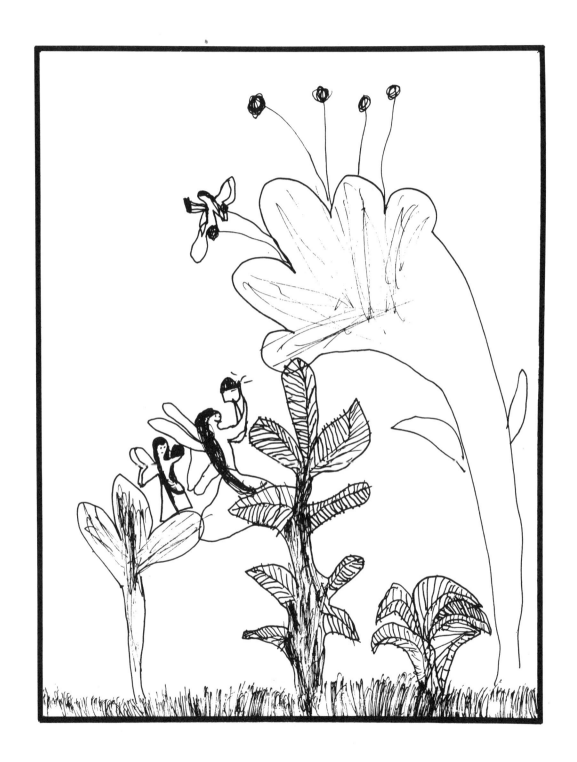

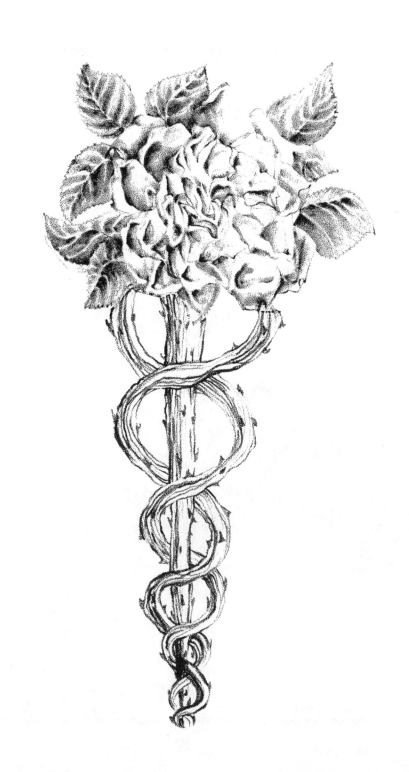

HYGIEIA

A WOMAN'S HERBAL

by Jeannine Parvati

Drawings by Tamara Slayton Glenn

Calligraphy by Quill Cleaver

Hygieia is the Greek Goddess of Health.

Hygieia is the Greek Goddess of Health.

Epione was her mother, Asclepius her father.

Her numerous siblings included Iaso (Goddess of Healing), which means "cure"; and Panacea or "all-healing".

She came from an illustrious family, to say the least. Her grandmother was Coronos, her grandfather, 'Apollo' himself.

On her father's side, that is, Epione was the daughter of Melops. Yet it is **Apollo** who is associated with healing and so it is his son Asclepius who carries on in this tradition.

Hygieia lived in a time when abandonment was very common. So it happened that her father, Asclepius was left to die as a baby. In the mountains a nanny-goat nursed him and his first caretaker was a dog. Eventually, a shepherd found him and delivered him to Cheiron, that marvelously wise centaur. Cheiron was half-man and half-horse, and a teacher to many youths. He was knowledgeable in the ways of herbs, and taught what he knew to Asclepius. When Ascelpius grew up, though he was an Oympian God, i.e. one of the head honchos on the gods and goddess' scene, he preferred to spend time **healing** - so humans began to worship him. They built shrines, places of healing, wherein the sick could come and be visited by Hygieia and her sisters.

Asclepius is said to have met his death by outraging Hades, the God of the Underworld. The story goes this way - one day, Asclepius, who was the first empiricist or true medicine man, noticed an ailing snake being treated by another snake. Hence the staff of Cadueses, the symbol of the medical profession with Apollo's staff being twined by two snakes. The ill snake dies - and then the other snake did an amazing thing. At least Asclepius hadn't ever seen his old teacher, Cheiron (who was the son of Old Chronos, father time himself) administer to the dead like this. The snake found an herb and placed the plant on the dead snake-friend. The dead snake revived! An herb to raise the dead! Asclepius then used the herb to bring a dead man back to life and for this he was killed. Hades showed Zeus how unfair it was to allow this kidnapping of his kingdom - for Hades ruled the world of the dead and didn't like to be cheated. Zeus threw a thunderbolt and that was the end of Asclepius. Now his father, Apollo, persuaded Zeus to see this punishment as a bit too severe, and so Asclepius was raised up into the stars. But before all this, he fathered the three healing sisters - Hygieia, Iaso, and Panacea.

Not as much is known about Hygieia as Asclepius, Apollo, etc. The male healers, at least in the Greek tradition, had better press than the women healers. This book, entitled Hygieia is our effort to change this.

And so it is to Hygieia that we draw our attention. She is the goddess within each of us who knows the grace of being healthy. We intone a chant to honor her, and our ancestors — ~O Coronus, Apollo, Melops, Epione, Acesis, Aegle, Iaso, Janiscus, Machaon, Panacea, Podalirius, and Hygieia~ bring us the blessing of health & the power to help heal our ~ sisters and brothers. ~

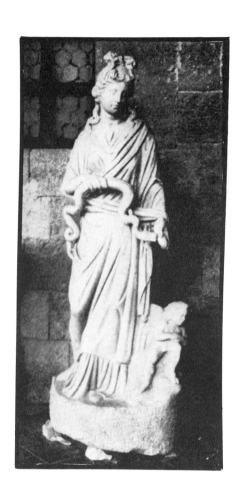 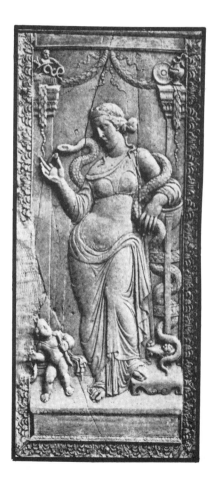

TABLE OF CONTENTS

INTRODUCTION

This little book is the chapter from a much bigger one on **Conscious Conception** *- and so it is written from a wholistic perspective on female sexuality and fertility. Being healthy is very important and so we thought we'd share this aspect first. The larger work, our opus, is now available through Freestone Publishing, our home business. Perhaps there is a benefactor amongst you - someone who will support us as we continue in our good work. Freestone Publishing Collective means, basically, responding to the muse through the perseverence of transiting Saturn and the help of some friends.*

Our thanks to the fathers of our children, Nancy Cleaver "Quill", clear calligrapher and alchemist; Baba Hari Dass, my yoga teacher; Dean and Mary Perlman who love my children when I write; Frederick Baker Thresh Publications for giving us encouragement just at the right time; Greenway, for opening up to me the world of book-making; and River, for keeping the business flowing; Candle, for giving me my woman soul; Bill Prange, who helps my fall into the Heart; Drake and Georgeanne of Guerneville Graphics; AND ALL OUR SISTERS WHO HAVE SHARED THEIR FAVORITE RECIPES TOWARDS HEALING OURSELVES THE HERBAL WAY. And our children deserve special thanking - Loi Caitlin, Zachary Tyler, Summer Glenn, Oceana Violet, and Cheyenne Coral. It is with much love that we dedicate this book to our mothers, VICKI O'BRIEN AND VERNA HARTLEY, for initiating us into womanhood.

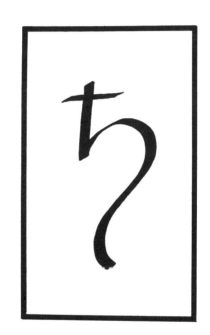

How Best to Use This Book

This book grew out of our need to be healthy and re-own the powers of naturally healing ourselves. In no way do we suggest that this book can replace a relationship that already exists between yourself and a healer/doctor. Oftentimes we do need help from someone else - and sometimes, we are startled into running to the doctor's office for a cure when the situation could best be handled at home. And nowadays, treatments given to women by medical men sometimes prove to be iatrogenic,* i.e., **causes** of even more serious diseases. This work is inspired not from any personal, negative reaction with western medicine but rather from my positive relationship with Self as Healer and herbs as the main tool in this process. My relationship with gynecology/obstetrics has been perfect. It is just time to share what I have learned these past years in handling diseases of women at home, and keeping my young family in good health. My three-year-old twin daughters, Cheyenne and Oceana, have but once needed doctoring, and never drugs. Their shining good health comes from **health consciousness** as a daily matter from way **before** their conception, with occasional herbal medicines and lots of affirmations. My eldest daughter, Loi, now 7½ years old, also is a beautiful example of what attention to diet, play/work, feelings, yoga, and love can be. Our regular "doctor" is named "Father Sun" and we visit him often to bathe in his glow; we also moon-bathe to honor the Mother. We grow our own vegetables and a few herbs and fruits - have our own goats for yogurt, cheese, etc. But more importantly, we bless our meals and imbibe our herbal teas with our thanks. This book is for wo/mankind - so that we can help one another realize the inherent bliss of being female.

The herbs have, somewhat **chauvinistically,** been called "she" and "her" rather than "it", and this is to remind the reader that by personifying our remedies, we bring a greater respect to the usage. This is also the tiny token towards bringing a balance back to the sexist English language, for language shapes our world-view and how we experience ourselves. One more use of language that may be confusing - that is the referral to douching as an external remedy, as has been done in herbals for many a century. The **vaginal canal** is considered **outside** of our bodies - **internal** treatments refer to **swallowing** herbal brews. I have left it as other herbalists describe douching, as an external application, though common sensing suggests that indeed a douche comes **into** oneself, and hence is an internal application of a remedy. Reflection on the reasons why herbalists have called douching an external application can prove illuminating. I'll leave this to you to consider.

* See **The Medical Nemesis by** Ivan Illich for a fuller discussion of this point.

*Wherever possible, I have included the Latin names so there will be no confusion. The already practicing herbalists will appreciate this, as well as the beginner. For those of you just entering into the world of herbs, you might skip the botanical names as you read so as not to further mystify yourself. Those names will become important if and when you purchase herbs, or look them up in a field identifier handbook, as you gather. I've found that reciting the Latin name when gathering herbs is akin to the liturgical chants - it's a way of pausing to thank the spirit of the plant as I take its life unto mine for purposes of healing. And as my foremothers have done, I never take all the herbs of a particular kind in any area so that the species will be able to propagate herself. One rule that my relatives taught me is to always skip the first plant I see and then gather the others in her vicinity of the same species. Practicing herbalists might like to use this rule, or create rituals of your own when in the "bush". There's even an etiquette for buying herbs in stores. Also, **smelling** the purchase is part of this. It is great fun to meet an herb, in a store, who I've been studying and know through her botanical name only - touching and smelling bring life to our relationship.*

*My father's family, the Colville Indians of Washington, are in part responsible for the interest I do have now in herbs. I remember my dad talking about how "white" men would disrespectfully ask for all the information on their medicinal and sacred herbs, so sometimes the wrong information would be given. With this in the back of my mind, I've had to take what other herbalists have written with a grain of salt. **Try it out in your own body** - home science, here and now. If it works, remember it, share your success and try again if the opportunity ever presents itself. Always listen to your own body over the words of any herbal book, including this one.*

*There's a power to language as well as with herbs. We purposely use the word "cunt" interchangeably with "vagina", etc., in an effort to discharge the fear of patriarchal punishments. WE can only be embarrassed by our anatomy and the English descriptive words by keeping them hidden, unused except in situations of anger, hysteria, and pain. "You cunt" can only hurt our little girls if we mystify the word by responding shamefully. Lenny Bruce said that if **the President** of the United States would introduce his cabinet as, "The nigger, Secretary of State, the spick, Dept. of Interior, etc., that prejudice would lose its vehicle for transmission. Let us not prejudice our daughters to their own bodies by being embarrassed by the word "cunt" ever again.*

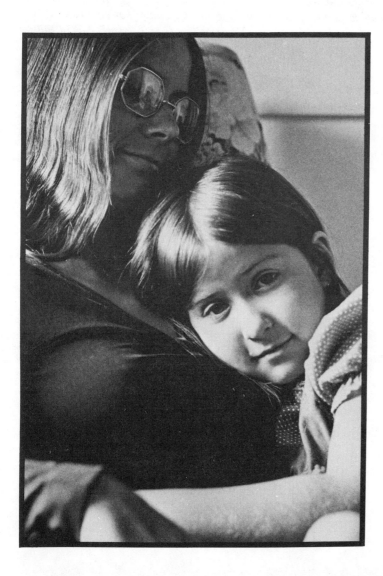

Quite purposefully, wherever possible, I have left the exact directions up to the reader on just how to go about using an herb. This is because of the emphasis on **relationship** *- learning from one another how best to heal. There are some general rules which help to focus the energy, though. And they are simple; I don't mean to mystify the procedure. Rather* **you** *discover from the plant herself how best to enter a healing relationship with one another. Herbs are powerful. They can do "miracles" if we but give them the respect and appreciation so rightfully theirs. Our suggested ritual for herb preparation is, (if possible), to gather them yourself, gently and with reverence for the spirit of the plant. Next best is to buy or be given the herbs from someone you trust, a favorite herb or health food store, and store them in clean, odorless glass and keep them in a cool dark place till needed. Boil your water, or make "Sun Tea" using the energy from the sun to steep the herbs for a much longer time outdoors in a sealed jar of pure water. Bring the tea pot* **to** *the prepared water, never the water to the teapot. A custom, or superstition - but as novices, each new mystifying ritual may bring later understanding and benefit on other levels than the cognitive or verbal level. As you place the herbs into the water, a prayer for the life-giving qualities of the plants may be evoked. They are transforming their energy into yours and we are deeply grateful. Once the herbal remedy is prepared, sit down comfortably with your cup of tea and slowly savor the brew. Just be with the herbs as they become a part of you. Do not take them with meals. A few hours before meals on an empty stomach is best, or at least wait an hour after food has been taken, ideally. Don't read, listen to the radio, or in any other way distract yourself from the herbal tea as you drink. Realize the specific purposes that are being served by this activity - for example, you want to stimulate menstruation as you sip on a soothing cup of chamomile so this is what you continually bring your mind to as you drink the herb. Yes, it is a meditation of sorts - the yoga of herbs. Tinctures, linaments, syrups and other herbal preparations are not included. So usually, wherever an herb is recommended as a drink or douche, an infusion or a steeped brew is fine. Experiment, watch, heal. It is the process of healing which must be accepted by you. Each of us has our own recipes for health and the procedures with herbs are but rituals of your own choosing. Let the plant be your guide.*

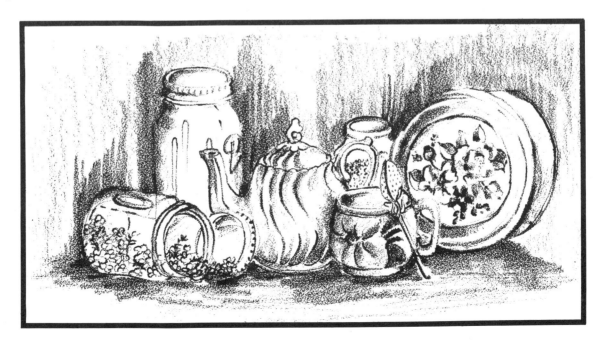

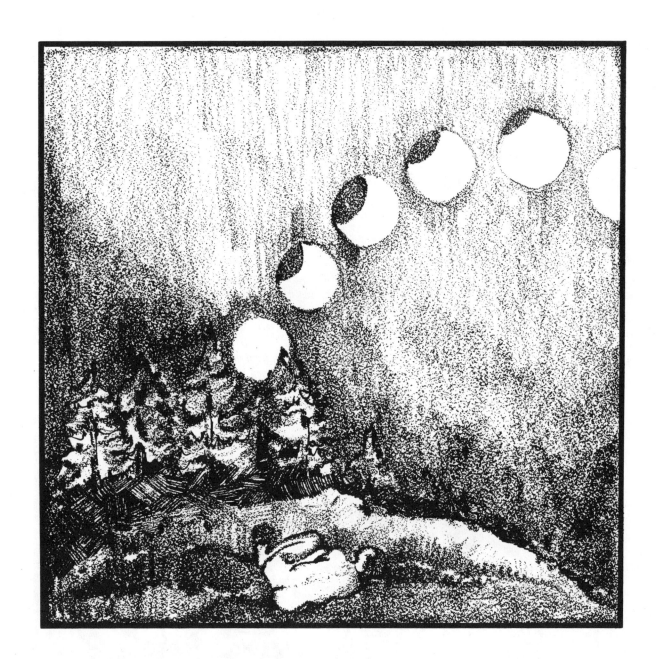

1

"On The Rag" & Other Menstrual Rituals

For You, Fertile Sister

Bleeding is part of being sexual. It is a time of grounding you with the Mother, our planet Earth. It is the announcement of fertility, and like any other aspect, has the possibilities of being as pleasurable as sex. What oftentimes gets in the way of experiencing menstruation as an **ecstatic renewal** are the images, our body fantasies, our cultural myths, and poor health. This book was written, in large part, to support cultural myths **celebrating** this particular aspect of female sexuality - namely, menstruation. The more obvious purpose, to share ways of being healthy via herbal **allies,** is our cover. And so, in regarding the menstrual process from a new-age perspective, we pause to **uncover** some fecund rituals which have renewed many of us.

It's no surprise that many women experience much discomfort, nay pain, when menstruating or just before. It **is** sad, I often feel, to realize another ovum has died - no baby, soon, to grow within. Feelings are intrinsically linked with the moon, and the menstruations. My **intuitions** show the link between this grieving and the organic, sensual pain of menstruation. Finally, I intuited that there was no need to create a dramatic upheaval in my home, in order to get my mate to "make me cry" (usually by being bitchy about **housecleaning**[1]). I could re-own those feelings myself, and have a good cry, letting go of the egg, the hope, with my tears. Then the blood flowed easier - and more pleasurably.[2] Lately I've come to see that my pleasure and pain are pretty much balanced - emphasis of avoiding one and seeking the other is wasteful of my energy. So - menstruation has become as beautifully satisfying of an experience as any other feminine expression of sexuality - i.e. pregnancy, childbirth, lactation, and most likely, menopause. Let me share my herstory - for probably like you, I once tucked my "soiled" sanitary napkins carefully in the garbage so that **no one would know** I was bleeding ... and the horror of "staining" my skirt in school... but let me begin, at the beginning, of my menstrual consciousness as a toddler in the 1950's.

(As an infant, too, there's a trace memory of my menstruating mom.)

She had a different smell - tummy much more soft - eyes softer too, when my mommy bled. The mother, I chose, was very open about menstruation.[3] My initiations into fertility are remembered as being nothing special, as important as any other aspect of living. Mom regarded her own blood dispassionately - as best as a little toddler could understand.[4] Images of blood coming out of female dogs in our neighborhood - the touching of my own first blood years later. Now I miss the lack of celebration and have since made up for it. After amenorrhea for three years (from the conception of my first daughter till over two years of breastfeeding), the subsequent return of menses was quite a party. In the midst of our hullabaloo, the phone rang and my 2 year old daughter, Loi, answered saying, "Hi! My mommy just got her period!!" The excitement has mellowed into a glow, now.

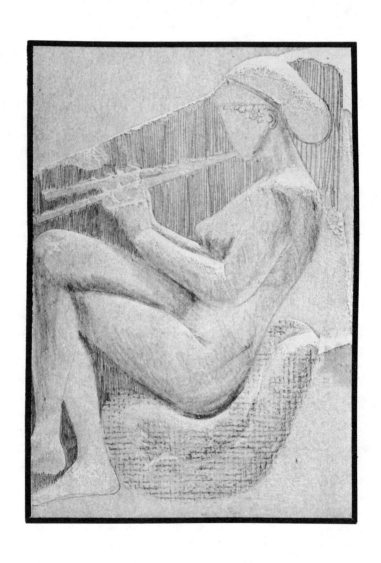

*Images of our dance collective - our full moon bleedings - our Witches' Dance on Halloween. Painting faces with our own blood. Giving the juices to favorite plants in my garden - squatting by those in need of minerals. Menstrual poems, menstrual weavings, bleedin'-heart songs. And women finally realizing that those sisters of ours, in "primitive" societies, who are banished during the menses, are actually enjoying a break from husbands and kids and the need to pretend that they are not menstruating. The tampax maiden in a white bikini is a powerful archetype. When I am menstruating, I am in a **very internal**[5] space. I do not remember my dreams as easily, and am intent upon the devotional nectar flowing from deep inside. With mindfulness upon the entire process of bleeding - breath bringing awareness of "letting go" - menstruation becomes a meditation. Emptying, emptying - letting go my life's juices as attention focuses on the center of my body. Yes, a cleansing - yet not in the way of implying fertile women as impure. Some menstruating sisters in other cultures are not allowed to touch food, or men. Come to think of it - I'm usually not hungry while bleeding, or horney. But I perceive the cleansing, called menstruation, as an opportunity for elimination of any negativity, toxins, pollutants, and/or energy blocks in my being. This perception is not with judgment. A menstruating woman, so often isolated in animistic cultures, (one's in which a time/temporality is quite different, more cyclic, than most of our consciousnesses as westerners), IS NOT seen as "bad" as many a male anthropologist would report, by implication. I know I live to retreat - at bleedings - to treat myself with the care of my sisters, and my Mother, our Earth. The menstruating women often gathered by the local source of water - **renewals** - and the sweat lodges - **purifications** - to chant together, massage, and share the way women do. Men seeing this, labelled us as "gossips": literally meaning "good woman friend". See how we have distorted our own words, our own rituals, our own experience . . . Bleeding grounds us. We are reminded, in all our humility, our connection to this planet and subsequent return to her womb. The blood reminds us of our mortality. There is no time to waste. Women will show the way to heal this Earth; we know the balancing of life and death, growing and letting go. Bleeding teaches us gentleness. How being slow and delicate in movement stills the mind. The monthly emptying opens us as channels - **to be filled once again without attachment**. Let us return to the tampax maiden in a white bikini as archetype. This image, as portrayed on billboard and hammered into consciousness of every school girl, does damage on many levels. First, the obvious one of using tampons, or any item sold to us by large industries, **that plugs us up**. But more on this later when we share some patterns and ideas for making your own menstrual pads. It is the effect on our power, as women, that concerns me here. When wearing a tampon (or natural sponge for that matter), one is less likely to retreat from the busy work-a-day world and carry on as usual. Actually, with plugs such as tampons, it's more accurate to say **the tampon is wearing you!** Women wear little red strings on their wrists to alert their friendship circle to their bleeding now - a reminder to be kind, and supportive of this altered state of consciousness. We lose power by pretending that bleeding is not occuring. We also pinch off our own energy by trying to hold in a bloated belly during menstruating. Girdles are our own shackles, pinching off a source of much power. Many yogis, after some time of pranyama and siddhis, develop pot bellies. This isn't to suggest you say, "ah! the hell with it"and let a paunchy tummy become a spare tire. What I am suggesting is that our body fantasy, in a vain attempt to be our current cultures' **pretty lady**, flatten our stomachs and flatten our power. The belly is the location of the **will**. This is one reason why many pretty ladies enjoy being pregnant so much - no need to flatten our will; bulging belly is O.K. under these circumstances. Presently my bleedings often come when I've **truly** let my desire to be pregnant go. Being as* *stubborn as I am, sometimes it takes some pretty dramatic rituals to bring on a bleeding. Oftentimes, a dream will signal the onset of menses - for years it was driving my red pick-up truck on the freeway and taking the Penngrove exit. Sure enough, I'd always awake to a first trickle of blood. Over the years of improving nutrition, meditation, and sexual relationships (I'm sure there are many more variables also), my menstrual flow has lightened up to being **just enough** to know I am fertile, yet not enough to need a pad, plug or other tool through which to soak up the experience. Sometimes, I know I am menstruating because my uterus feels as if some velvet hand was massaging me from the inside-out. Or I will sense the wetness between my legs, via smell, as blood. Rarely do I bleed longer than a day anymore.[6] I believe this comes from giving my full attention to the process - not in any effort to "reduce" or shorten bleeding - this has been a side-effect and one that personally I enjoy; makes squatting in the garden for the major part of the flow plausible when it lasts only an hour or so, retreating to the sauna for the remainder of the day/night. I have also arranged my life (with the exception of speaking gigs and midwifery so that if I am menstruating, I don't "go to work". Re-write your own life-script to include the experiencing of menstruation as a sexual, cleansing, and liberating (see Appendices) process that is but one of the many gifts for being female. And then share your nourishing rituals with sisters everywhere. We are all in this together.*

*There seems no dearth of controversy about the amount or **any** menstrual blood as a sign of women's health. In **Survival in the 21st Century**, MENSTRUATION does not even occur in an aquarian body. Or in other words, the bleeding is a sign that the old way of eating (which is any diet except breath, sprouts and fruit) is still in effect. Emmenagogic herbal teas are necessary for those of us who do eat other things than the above - who are fertile (and a bit toxic perhaps) and want to get the flow going. I personally find judgments such as these helpful only to the extent that I am inspired to live more harmoniously with my world, with food being simple, and prana (divinely-charged air) being my most conscious "meal". If I take such a statement, and reflect a copious flow of menstrual blood as indication of being very unhealthy, "old age" or not aquarian, and feel bad about this - then eat a little more cheesecake to make myself feel better . . . well, you can see that this isn't helpful. I'm suspicious somewhat of all this androgynous mythology springing up to the extent that it denies women experiences of their sexuality - i.e. menstruation. How can we make the move towards more balanced living (androgyny) if our most feminine experiences are labelled "unhealthy"?*

*The amount of menstrual blood is also traditionally associated with the amount of sexual intercourse. Here I found that the definition of sexual intercourse is inclusive of sexual unions in thought, imagination, fantasy, dreams, creative (artistic process) as well as the desire and physical relationship of **loving**. Victoria Woodhall, a name every feminist prides herself upon knowing well, wrote that "the curse" befalls only the animals that indulge in sex for purposes other than procreation. She is obviously a child of the Victorians as she writes, "Where is the female animal that wastes her life away at every changing moon?" She concurs with many other learned folk that menstruation is a loss of precious body fluid. In the Hindu health mythologies, **the ojas**, a precious fluid released at sexual intercourse by the woman, is very vital to the woman's subtle body as well as the physical and it's best not to waste them for a few seconds of ecstasy - save it for the eternal bliss of union with God. In the Karezza Method of non-seminal intercourse, one propenent (a woman M.D., Alice Stockham) suggests the woman retain her vital fluids and **not** orgasm. The element of containment and transformation is a common thread between menstruation and orgasm (ovulation) on this weaving of a woman's soul.*

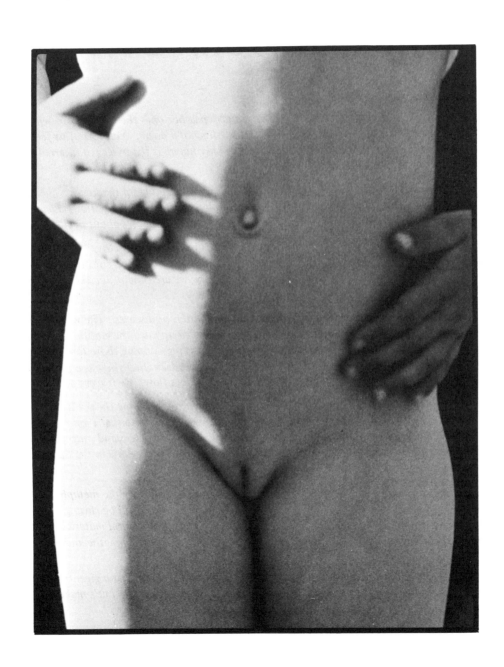

Making Your Own

There's an art to bleeding - as in everything else. The sanitary pad becomes the canvas onto which you pour the paint of your being. Many a flow has begun with the birthing of a poem. Yet, lots of us feel the creative flow is stopped up (especially just before our periods are due) and my hunch is the usages of internal pads and even natural sponges has lots to do with this.

Physiologically, tampons etc., are non-discriminating in their job of soaking up the juices. This means **all** our fluids - not just blood. How many of us feel dried out completely after a menstruation? Please, don't be afraid of your own juiciness - again the "discharges" are messages from our bodies about cyclical fertility.

Psychologically, (and I realize categorizing experiences of human-ness is only relative to the Truth; that we have no separation between mind/body), with tampons etc., there's a block in freely flowing - the release is only partial. We are also hiding something very important about how we are - the soul essences are also being soaked up to be discarded with yesterday's rubbish and hopes for a baby.

Emotionally, keeping the flow inside, and hidden, maintains all kinds of diseases. The worry, fear and other non-appreciations and acceptances of how we are each moment, is bottled up until the emotional body can manifest this bound energy in other ways. That's why a good cry is often so relieving - unplug those tampons, loosen those throats* (cervixes = **neck** is the translation of this Latin word - and it does seem that there is a physio-psycho-emotional connection between our cervixes and our necks), so let the juices flow! Be it tears or blood.

Spiritually, when a tampon is wearing me, (or I think that I'm effectively hiding the reality of menstruation from the 'outer' world) the illusion of separateness is maintained. How can I believe that I am merely a skin-encapsulated ego, apart from all, **when bleeding** and feeling the flow go down my legs and onto the Earth. How I can feel "unique" when in the sweat lodge with my many bleeding sisters. We are one in the Spirit, in the Sun, and in the Blood.

Firstly, choose your material well - the menstruation metaphor involves deeply the **metaphor on the material**. Begin with texture - how your pad would feel on your cunt. Remember that you will be rinsing it often and perhaps sterilizing it upon occasion (for those believers in the Germ Theory). A **natural** material cannot be stressed enough. Wearing synthetic (nylon underwear, for example), doesn't let your vagina breathe and 'chapped lips',

* There is a political concern in purchasing pre-packaged sanitary napkins. We support a gigantic industry that perpetuates images of powerless, pretty ladies - and equates "whiteness" with purity. Let's make our own!

*sore vulva, and/or vaginal infections sometimes are the result. Only cotton, wool, silk. Note what color you feel like wearing. I notice that I wear more reds in my dreams during menstruation, so a piece of red flannel material seemed appropriate. No one said you **have** to wear white. No surgery's been performed, we aren't playing doctor. An image of a purple, red, gold, silver mandala appliqued to the center of your menstruation pad just appeared. Think how much soul force you'd be imbuing the flow to wear such a pad! Natural sponges are advantageous over tampons for many reasons. First, it is reusable and therefore ecological. Secondly, we aren't supporting a huge and no doubt, polluting industry when we rinse out our own sponges.[8] This is a good way to get "in touch" with your periods. Handling your sponge and blood helps to discharge lots of our self-disgust, so inculcated by media, myths and poor health. You have an opportunity to **smell** your blood - a very powerful experience when the cerebral cortex is not involved* - and even **taste** your blood as Germaine Greer prescribed for all you who consider yourselves sexually liberated feminists. The handling of our own secretions will prepare you for the sometimes bloody experiences of childbirth, and other crises. Blood will cease to "freak you out".*

Equally as rare is the experience of fertility without menstruation. That is, there is cyclical ovarian function but no bleeding. Many philosophers and nutritionists testify to this possibility. Some agree that the menstrual blood is highly toxic (due to the presence of various acids and heightened leucocyte content). Then we have the middle of the road experts saying that most often when menses stops, it's for reasons other than healthful ones, like "malnutrition". While I found the male authors discoursing about the toxicity of menstruation, the female writers concerned themselves with just what women actually do. When an Apache woman fails to menstruate but is not pregnant, she is considered diseased with what is called "blood is in her". A treatment administered by a medicine wo/man consisted of making a tea from the chipped branch which had been struck by lightening and blessing it with sacred pollen. A Cahuilla woman who doesn't agree with the literature about the evils of bleeding, and desires her menses, goes to seek help. One woman visited a medicine man in California who waited until the next new moon. He then inserted a long stick up his nose till it bled, collected it and then rubbed the blood with his hands into the abdomen of the amenorrhea-striken woman. She menstruated the next day. Of course, I would too if it meant someone would stick a stick into his nose! I once watched Rolling Thunder doctor a terrible headache. He literally excited the pain and with the aid of his power (an eagle feather), sucked it out of the woman's head. Then he threw it up and she was recovered. The smell of protecting herbal smoke covered us all. I thought then that I too would give up my headache rather than have anyone suck violently the top of my head and then vomit. So it is with menstruation rituals; we have many choices and ways to heal. There are many herbs which aid in the promotion of menstruation. Several of the major ones are cleansing ones (blood purifiers). The following collections are grouped into emmenagogues and menstrual remedies. But please recall that herbs can be used as band-aids too. Just treating the symptoms, without curing the underlying trouble, is temporary at best and may mask a more serious health crisis.

** The sense of smell is a more primal one - being the only sense to directly go into the Limbic System of the brain rather than mediated through our "thinking". Our deepest feelings, and memories, are best stimulated by odors. Using feminine "hygiene" sprays (actually **iatrogenic** and to be avoided), confuses not only ourselves but lovers as well. We invite you, the reader, to share your menstrual rituals as personal stories with us. We won't promise a **personal** response to each one - just know that we will be reading them and valuing them whole-heartedly; might publish some in our Conscious Conception book, if you say it's O.K.*

PATTERN for MAKING YOUR OWN

The most important aspect of this process ~ "making your own" ~ is the sense of self-worth and appreciation you bring to this ritual. Creating a receptacle for your blood is a positive affirmation of your femaleness and is to be celebrated. ~

suggested materials

soft cloth, rags, velvet, calico, muslin, satin

1" wide elastic

velcro ~ self-adhesive tape

cotton batting or sponge

herbs: pennyroyal, cinnamon, peppermint, raspberry, chamomile, & so on.

the pad

① Take a piece of cloth approx. 10" x 15", fold long edges in 2" & then into the middle like this ~

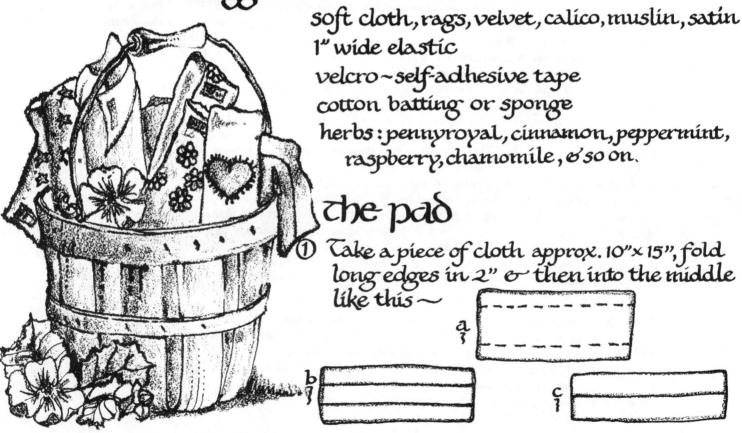

② Turn edges under to form tabs, like this~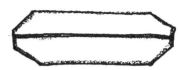

③ Sew edges down. Attach velcro to inside edges.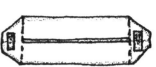

You now have a cloth envelope in which to
stuff cotton batting or sponge, and herbs
of your choosing.

the belt

① Measure hips and double this length. Take a piece of cloth
4" wide & your length. Fold in half, sew along edge &
turn inside out.

② Insert elastic and herbs.

③ Attach ends together, forming a circle.

④ Attach other half of self-adhesive tape to outside of belt
and match up.

It works best
to have at least two pads,
so one can be drying while
you wear the other.

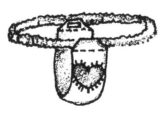

for cleaning,
remove cotton batting,
rinse cloth & dry. Or
remove sponge, rinse
in hot water & place
in clean pad.~

happy bleeding!

Carnivores & Menses

The natural tendency among women to fast or not eat any meat is rooted in many tribes of peoples during menses.

Menstruation was much less common an experience with the native women here in North America. Either a woman was pregnant, or nursing. Sometimes she may be sterile and not menstruating at all. But it was not so often that a woman was bleeding **every month** the year round. And so, the taboos which sprung up around a woman's menstruation, were not enforced as an everyday thing.

In some worlds, a menstruating woman is called upon for special uses in hunting. The Mandans of North Dakota, for example. Here, women who are bleeding are in great demand for eagle catching. But in most places, women avoided eating meat and participating in any way with the carnivore game. The Yokut believed that eating meat when menstruating would make a woman sterile. For the Cocopah, fish was taboo for the same reason. Hunters guarded against any contact with a menstruating woman. Some would lose their power if they were healers also.

Sex During Menses

With Masters and Johnson, other sex experts, being quoted all over the literature about sex during menses as a decongestive and relaxing aid, the notion of a taboo for the young women menstruating **and** fucking simultaneously doesn't hold much ground. However, the possibility of conception occurring then is so often confirmed that the taboo for its contraceptive purposes alone is worth revising.

I can see the prohibition about meat being valid during menstruation as another metaphor for indulgences in the flesh. Eating meat means the inevitable elimination of the indigestable parts during the bloody flow - having sex then may also signify the later birthing of a baby. It has been thought by many women and cultures that this relationship (see our dark-lady-inclination-of-the-night) is **powerful**.

This prohibition was much supported by the native American people. Some say that this was not to usurp man's power and to protect all manner of things such as skills, the hunt, good weather - and some report that this was also considered a birth control taboo. The Navajo, Hopi, Omaha and Havasupai among others believe that conceptions are most likely to occur during menstruation. The Navajo men, must be on top while making love with a menstruating woman or else he runs the risk of pregnancy himself!

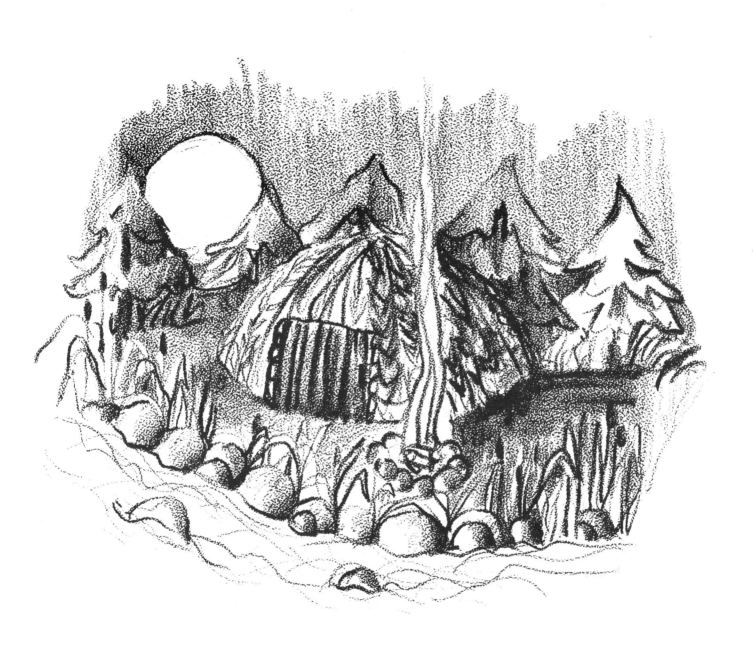

An emmenagogue promotes the menstrual flow. They range from the mild 'chamomile' used by Spanish-speaking women in the Americas for centuries to the stronger 'cohoshes' that work directly on the uterine lining. The herbs included are not intended as abortifacients, i.e. they will not terminate a pregnancy in the dosages recommended.

*One of the most often "anonymous" phone calls I receive comes as a question. "Which herb can I drink to bring on my period?" Behind this question oftentimes is a fear, fear·of being pregnant. Herbal abortions are not necessarily any easier than a technological one - in fact, sometimes they are more difficult. If the caller is **worried**, yet not pregnant, her period can be hung up due to the interconnection of feelings and bodily functions. The hypothalamus is next to the pituitary gland, our seat of emotions affecting the master gland for reproductive systems. Emmenagogues are a great help here. They can help you relax enough to flow. But let us not use these herbs like pills; use herbs always as tools to understanding ourselves. Meditating on the mythology of the herbal emmenagogue while you use the plant will bring you closer to the spirit of healing. We can make many friends with emmenagogic herbs to use if needed; to help aid the menstrual flow, the de-toxification, and the celebration. My favorite aspect of Don Juan's work as a Yaqui medicine man was the making of plant allies Emmenagogues are women's gentlest allies.*

*There can be a yoga to using herbs for health, for soul-making, and for the good of us all. The following herbs are shared as an **incomplete** search for female allies in the plant world. These lists are meant to be absorbed over long periods of time. As you need a remedy, the information will become alive in the **using**. I've purposely incorporated mythology, legends, and stories about many herbs so as to keep the healing properties in perspective. (Diseases are but messages from the Gods.) Botanical classification (the Latin words) are reported for the more serious herbologists amongst you, and to avoid a mistake. As for the herbs listed, I chose the ones with whom I had a basic resonance. I knew the herb already and had used it on myself, or knew of someone who had, or liked the P.R. from other herbalists about the particular herb I'm writing about. Remember to always, **all ways**, check it out in your own body. More on this aspect later (which herb is right for me?) in the discussion of intuition and radiesthesia, astrology, tarot, etc. in our forth coming book on **Conscious Conception**. No one is a greater expert about you and your health, than **you**! Home science.*

*A few words about **how** to use herbs must be said. Herbs are powerful. They can do "miracles" if we but give them the respect and appreciation so rightfully theirs. Our suggested ritual for herb preparation is, (if possible), to gather them yourself, gently and with reverence for the spirit of the plant. Next best is to buy or be given the herbs from someone you trust, a favorite herb or health food store, and store them in clean, odorless glass and keep them in a cool dark place till needed. Boil your water, or make "Sun Tea" using the energy from the sun to steep the herbs for a much longer time outdoors in a sealed jar of pure water. Bring the tea pot **to** the prepared water, never the water to the teapot. A custom, or superstition - but as novices, each new mystifying ritual may bring later understanding and benefit on other levels than the perceptual or cognitive/verbal level. As you place the herbs into the water, a prayer for the life-giving qualities of the plants may be evoked. They* *are transforming their energy into yours and we are deeply grateful. Once the herbal remedy is prepared, sit down comfortably with your cup of tea and slowly savor the brew. Just be with the herbs as they become a part of you. Do not take them with meals. A few hours before meals on an empty stomach is best or at least wait an hour after food has been taken, ideally. Don't read, listen to the radio, or in any other way distract yourself from the herbal tea as you drink. Realize the specific purposes that are being served by this activity. For example, you want to stimulate menstruation as you sip on a soothing cup of chamomile, so this is what you continually bring your mind to as you drink the herb. Yes, it is a meditation of sorts - the yoga of herbal birth control.*

One more word on abortion - since writing this chapter (now almost a decade ago), many have told me that my words have helped mothers keep their babies. Whenever I hear of a woman aborting her baby, I receive the news with my heart to the ground. If any of my readers cannot wait to read **Conscious Conception,** *you can write for more information to: Feminists For Life of America*
1918 Upton Avenue North
Minneapolis, Minnesota 55411

Here are my favorite herbs for menstruation rituals ~

the emmenagogues.

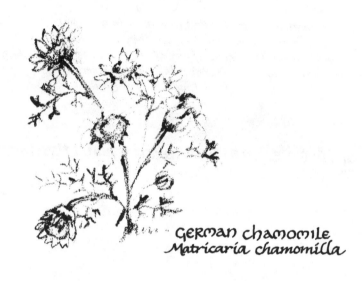

GERMAN chamomile
Matricaria chamomilla

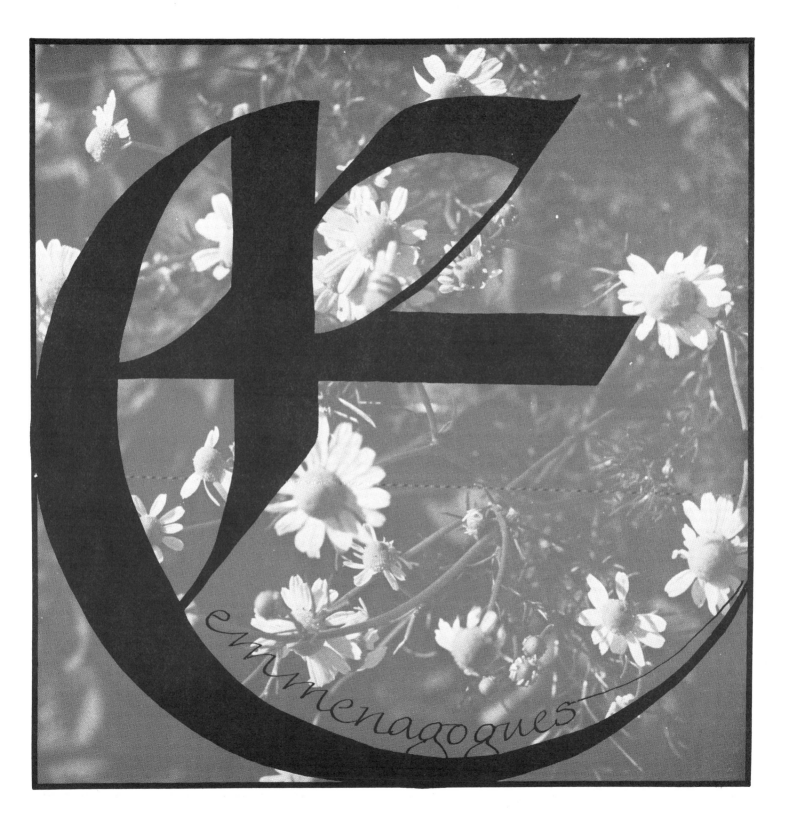

emmenagogues

Emmenagogues

Aloe

Aloe fruticosa. As an emmenagogue, the dose is from 5 - 20 centigrams for a tonic effect, and from 30 centigrams to one gram for a purgative effect. It should not be used by people with piles as it acts on the large intestine, drawing blood to that area. It is best used as a carminative. It is extremely bitter to taste. The Indians call aloe "the wand of heaven". Legend says it's the only plant to come directly from the Garden of Eden. Used sometimes to increase the menstrual flow; its main use is as a first aid for burns. Also, it is used with white vinegar to cure falling hair by applying to the scalp. Let it set for a few minutes before shampooing.

Angelica

Archangelica officinalis umbelliferae. Important! Do not confuse this with poison hemlock, of the same family. Take 30 grains (about 3/8 of a tsp.) at a time of the root powder. It's reported to bring on menstruation and to expel the placenta. Angelica astropurpurea. "Dead nettle". "Masterwort". This has the same uses. It's old German name is "root of Holy Ghost". The Laplanders chew the root like tobacco and believe it lengthens life. The root is sweet smelling and thought to be the scent of angels, hence its name. Carried, it protects against infections and other evil spirits. Anna Riva suggests you sprinkle it about the house for the same purpose.

Balm

See "Infertility".

Basil

Ocimum minimum or Ocium basilicum. "Sweet Basil". Once used often in white magic. A decoction of basil with honey and a dash of nutmeg is reported to ease childbirth and expel the placenta. Easy to grow and good for bringing a fever down in a baby. Do this by giving a tepid or cooling bath of steeped basil. The Jews hold sprays of basil in their hands for strength during religious fasts. The tea taken hot is good in suppressed menses. It has been regarded as a sacred herb in India, of Vishnu and Krishna. It's planted in the home garden to be revered by the entire family. Hindus invoke the powers of protection and bring fertility with this herb. Wreaths have been found, in Egyptian burial chambers in the pyramids, made of basil. It also promotes the production of mother's milk. According to Dr. Fleming, Indian women of Chile used Basil to relieve the pains of childbirth. Medicas, spanish speaking herbalists, used this herb, known to them as Albica, for curing menstrual pains, morning sickness, and expelling the afterbirth. She's known lastly as a Talismanic charm. The youths of Sicily in our time wear a sprig of Basil behind their ear to denote the fact that they are of marriageable age and romantically inclined. Kept open in a bowl, the aroma tends to make the occupants of the room "happy and gay".

Bay Laurel Also used as an emmenagogue.

23

Black Cohosh *Cimicifuga racemosa "macrotys". She is used for pelvic diseases. See "Cycle Herbs".*

Blue Cohosh *Caulophyllum thalictroides L. "squaw root". Aside from its emmenagogic properties, it can be used to stem an excessive flow. It helps to regulate one's menses. Used by Menominee, Potawatomi, and Meskwaki Indians, Cohosh is an Algonquian name which has been applied to other herbs as well. Wiener reports the Chippewas used a strong decoction as a contraceptive or for ovarian and womb trouble. She treats leukorrhea, and increases menstrual flow.*

Blue Vervain *See Verbena under "Cycle Herbs".*

Camphor *Cinnamomun camphora. Ancient herbalists ascribed great emmenagogic properties to camphor. Homeopathic remedies are negated by exposure to its vapors. It is also used for hysterical complaints, and for "irritating conditions of the sexual apparatus" says J. Rose. Arabians used it to lessen sexual desire. Use it with care if at all.*

Catnip *Nepeta cataria L., "catmint". The plant is used to bring on delayed menstruation. It **increases** the flow. It's an ancient medicine for babies and young children for expelling wind, or curing hiccups and stomach spasms (colic). It's a pain reliever and nerve soother. Since medieval times it has been used to summon up fierceness during battle by chewing it.*

Chamomile *Matricaria chamomilla, "German chamomile". Anthemis nobilis, "Roman chamomile" compositae. A very fragrant herb, it has a sweet apple scent. It's very useful for female complaints. South American and Mexican women have used it as an emmenagogue. It's just wonderful as an herbal bath for you and especially for your baby. One of the ideal calming herbs for your wearlsome toddlers, it is also good for hysterical complaints. It is reported to increase the menstrual flow. Also called "manzanilla". After a birthing, Chicana midwives give a tea of this to promote a peaceful sleep in the mother, and through her colostrum, to the new-born baby. Hung up around the house, Riva suggests Chamomile will protect against lightning.*

Cinnamon *Cinnamomum zeylanicum, "oil of cassia". Hermann writes, "It stimulates the uterus, menstruation, and uterine hemorrhages." In Egypt it was used for embalming and for witchcraft. It was once more valuable than gold. In medieval Europe it was used as an aphrodisiac. "Upon inhalation, the oil is reported to act as a sexual stimulant to the female", states J. Rose. The leaves were used to decorate the ancient Roman temples. "Laurus cinnamomun". The Arabians valued the bark and used the oil to anoint the sacred vessels used in religious ceremony. Only the priests were allowed to gather cinnamon bark. Folkard reports that the ancients used the flowers in distilled water as a love potion. I use the bark to flavor our warm apple cider on winter nights.*

Cimifuga Rt. *See Black Cohosh; "Cycle Herbs".*

Corydalis   *Because this herb looks like Aristolochia clematitus, corydalis has been regarded as an emmenagogue. It is also said to have the same properties as fumitory, says Hermann.*

Cotton Root   *Gossypium herbaceum. A great friend of reproduction, she is used to hasten or initiate childbirth, contract the uterus in cases of suppressed or obstructed menses, and also to remove sexual weariness. Two ounces of the powdered bark to a pint of boiling water. Let sit a few minutes. To be used when freshly brewed only. May be taken several times a day.*

Creeping Thyme o Thyme   *Thymus serpyllum Labiatae. The "women's herb" of Central Europe and the Alps in folk medicine. It is excellent taken hot for suppressed or obstructed menses. Thymus vulgaris will produce perspiration when taken hot. Also it is called "Mother of Thyme". This herb was given in folk medicine to pregnant women in the Alps. It makes a good bath for sickly children.*

Dittany of Crete   *Dictamamus. In the twelfth book of the Aenead, Venus goes to Crete to gather Dittany. The ancients regarded it as an emmenagogue.*

Double Tansy   *See Tansy.*

Larkspur   *Delphinium ajacis or D. consolida, "Delphinium". She is an emmenagogue, especially in its wild form. Hermann compared her with Asconde. All plants contain alkaloids which can be poisonous. She is only rarely used for internal use for humans. She is used to kill head lice, nits, and vermins. Seeds are used as an insecticide.*

Lavendar   *Lavendula spica and Lavendula vera. Abiatae. It has been said that sprinkled upon one's head helps keeping chaste. My friend, Nan, the Midwife, always wears it to a birthing. "It helps the energy", she says. Gather the potent flowers when they are newly open. The whole plant is medicinal. She is a nervine, used for hysteria. She is great in herb pillows. Her perfume was used to scent a room by the Romans to prepare for childbirth. They used her also to promote the menses and deliver the placenta. A decoction of the flower buds can be used as a douche for leùkorrhea. Lavender flowers, or* **Alucena,** *aids a newborn in ridding his body of mucous. The medica would trace a cross with the dried, crushed leaves, over hot coals, to fill the room with this scent during birthing.*

Licorice Root   *See "Infertility".*

Life Root   *She is a female regulator. Muhr says she is good for promoting menstrual flow. Ingredient for formula number 195.*

Little Mallow *Malva parviflora L. The leaves have been used to induce perspiration and the menstrual flow. The marshmallow is used to increase the milk of mothers, speed delivery, ease the pain of urination and gonorrhea and the roots and seeds can be boiled in white wine and massaged into breasts to ease swelling.*

Marigold *Calendula officinalis. It was considered an emmenagogue in older times, and now in the U.S. Formerly, an extract of marigold, crushed blossoms in alcohol, diluted with water, was used for carcinomas of the breasts and of the womb. Several writers have recommended it for obstructions of the uterus.*

Marjoram *Origanum marjorana. "Sweet marjoram". Its name means "joy of the mountain". It is excellent for suppressed menstruation. No Italian salad is complete without a handful of leaves of marjoram. Taken hot as a tea, it will promote perspiration as well as increase the flow of menstruation.*

Masterwort *Heracleum lanatum. "Madnep", "Youthwort", "Cow parsnip". It is used for suppressed menstruation when the flow is scanty and painful.*

Mexican Tea *Chenopodium ambrosiodes. "Wormseed", "Jerusalem Tea", "Spanish Tea", "strong-scented pigweed". In New Mexico, it is used to promote menses and also to reduce a heavy and painful flow. It has also been used for after-birth pains.*

Mint *See Aphrodisiac Herbs.*

Montana Totentosa *This is an emmenagogue that is used by the Zapotec Indians of Mexico.*

See "Cycle Herbs", (other chapter).

Motherwort *See "Cycle Herbs".*

Origanum *Origanum vulgare. "Wild marjoram", "Mountain mint". This is good for suppressed menstruation or urine. It is also good for the "itch". Steep a heaping tablespoon in a pint of boiling water for 30 minutes. Dip a cloth in and apply as a heating compress to a sore throat, bind loosely with a dry cloth, then cover with oiled silk, says Kloss.*

Pennyroyal HEDEOMA PULLEGIADIES *"Squaw mint". An infusion of dried or fresh leaves and flower tops were used by the Rappahanock Indians to bring on a delayed menstruation. She is the American Pennyroyal that possesses this emmenagogic properties. Taken with blue cohosh, five days before bleeding is due, she promotes the flow and facilitates the regulation of menses.*

Pennyroyal *Mentha puelgium* "Squaw mint". If troubled with suppressed or scanty menses, take 1 or 2 cupfuls hot at bedtime along with a hot foot bath several days before expected. It will relieve nausea, but should not be taken by pregnant women, says Kloss. The oil is abortive and potentially fatal to the mother as well as the fetus. A menstrual regulator used by the Indians, it will increase the flow. It is also used for uterine exhaustion following childbirth and uterine ulcers. I repeat, it should not be taken by pregnant women. Take 2 tablespoons before meals, 3 times daily. It is also specific for the ovaries. Kloss says that, tied to your bedpost, she is said to increase brain power, and to make one aware and alert. Also if carried when traveling by water, pennyroyal is said to prevent seasickness.

Purple Stem Angelica *Angelica atropurpurea L.* "Masterwort". The roots are used to stimulate suppressed menses. See Angelica.

Ragwort See "Cycle Herbs".

Red Cedar, Eastern See "Cycle Herbs".

Red Sage See Sage.

Rue, Common *Ruta graveolens. Rutaceae.* An infusion of this plant has been used to promote delayed menstruation. She will increase the flow. The witches in medieval times used it as a stimulative and an irritant drug for female disorders. The oil is a poisonous abortifacient. Large doses can cause nerve derangements. An infusion of the herb is used for hysteria. She is the only herb Mohammed is known to have blessed. This herb in Iraq is eaten with raisins to overcome fears. She treats pain in pregnancy (caution). She is also used for faulty menstruation and congestion of the womb. Small doses, only, should be used. It is also known as the "Herb of Repentance" or the "Herb of Grace" and those who have a bit of Rue and sincere sorrow for any wrong caused another are assured full forgiveness both in this world and any others, reports Anna Riva. Also, to hold a love, take her, or his, right shoe, and write your name on its sole. Then fill the shoe with rue and hang it from a red cord from your bed. Your lover will be there as long as the shoe continues to hang.

Russian Thistle *Salsola kali L.* "Tumbling thistle", "Saltwort". This herb has been used to promote menstrual flow and to decrease water retention in the body.

Sage *Salvia officinalis.* Sage foot soaks are great when menstruating. Rubbing the sage over the genitals helps bring on delayed menses. It is also used to suppress mammary secretion, or "dry up milk", and also as a tonic after childbirth, in the case of the stillborn. She is excellent with **mugwort** and yarrow for promoting

27

menstruation. Drink 2 to 3 cups daily; again, the afternoon and evening are the best time. Red sage increases the menstrual flow, (Salvia Colorata), and is listed by Kloss as an aphrodisiac. She will also check this tendency if too profuse. She's used also, with beneficial effect, for the female organs where the pelvis is small. A bit of sage absorbs any ill fortune which may enter the home when hung over the doorway. She is used by both males and lesbians to induce lust in another woman, by pulverizing with a mortar and pestle some sage into a powder, placing her in a small glass vial and leaving her in the sun's rays for at least 10 days. Then, place some, just a pinch, under your tongue when you meet a woman you desire. Riva reports that it will make you irresistible to the human female. The spell is best performed on the day before the woman starts her menses.

Sagebrush, Big Artemisia tridentata. "Wormwood". A poultice was made and placed on the stomach to induce menstruation. Artemisia Absinthium. "Wormwood". This species is used for leukorrhea. Steep a heaping teaspoon in a cup of boiling water for 30 minutes. Drink 1 to 2 cups daily.

Sumac Berries See "Cycle Herbs".

Summer Savory See herbs for "Infertility".

Tansy Tanacetum vulgare L. "Golden Buttons". The flowery tops were used to promote menstruation, says Vogel. Kloss said it is good for leukorrhea. In olden days, tansy was used for hysteric disorders. In the 17th century, it was mixed with powdered ivory and coral and used for uterine discharge. It is safest used only externally. It is a dangerous abortifacient. Kloss reports that it increases the menstrual flow.

Thyme Thymus vulgaris. From the medieval ages, we've used this herb for female complaints: to induce menstruation, provoke abortion, and to ease pain in genitals and hips. It's a reliable nervine and excellent for nightmares. It can be used as a bath herb and for children, in frequent and small doses. It is also used in treating scabies, and will increase the menstrual flow.

Verbena See "Cycle Herbs".

Water Avens Geum rivale. "Te del Indio". This was used by the Flambeau Ojibway Indians; they used the wild species, Geum macrophyllum. An infusion was made, and after heating it and skimming the infusion, the women drank this as a powerful emmenogogue.

Water Pepper   Polygonum punctatum, "Smart weed". This is an emmenagogue and is a best known remedy for pain in the bowels, and for ulcers. It is also used as a mouth wash for sore mouth in nursing mothers.

Wild Carrot   See "Aphrodisiacs".

Wild Ginger   See "Temporary Sterility".

Wintergreen   See "Cycle Herbs".

Yarrow   See "Cycle Herbs".

Yew   Tauxus baccata. This is listed by Hermann as an emmenogogue. It is very acrid bitter and nauseus, however. Use the bark and the leaves.

"menstrual blood under Kirlian photography looks like a human fetus."

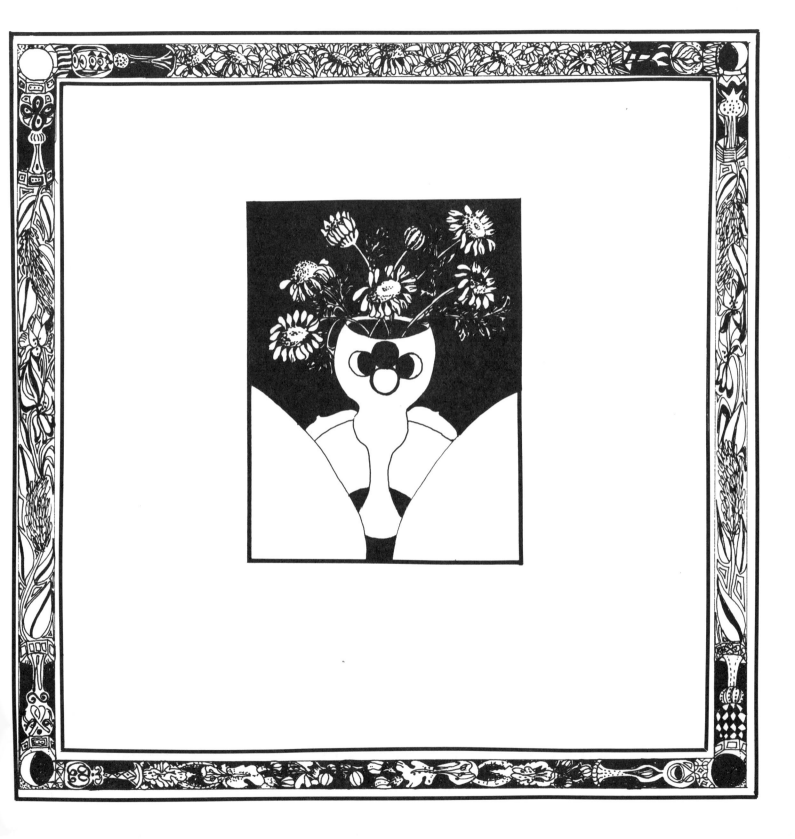

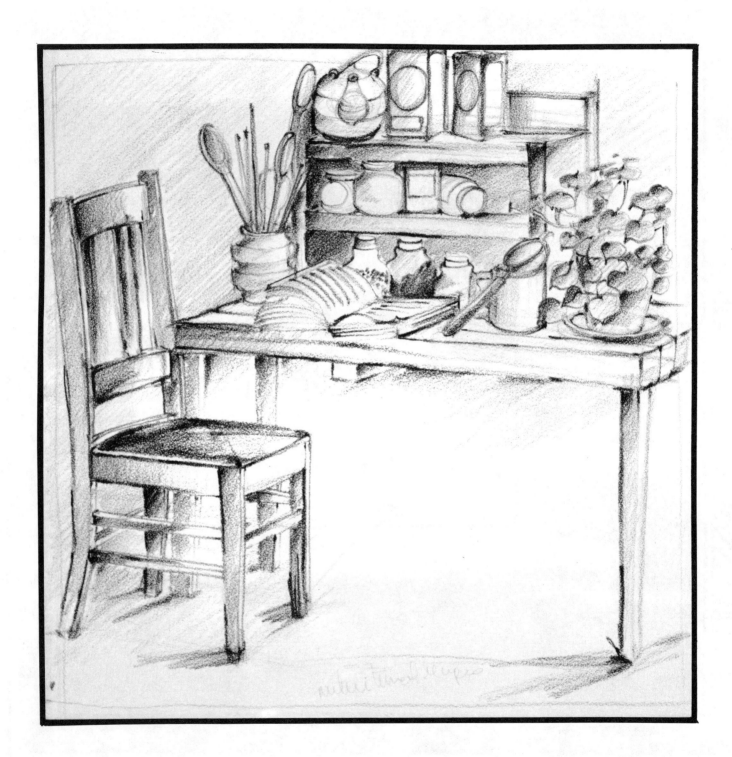

Nutritional Herbal Recipes

Good basic teas to replace needed minerals and fluids for menstruating (and nursing) women are the IRON TEA and CALCIUM TEA. The feeling will be of extra energy and peacefulness if drunk for several months at a time. And in our culture, because we have less babies and more periods, they are especially vital.

Iron Tea: Equal parts of: Yellow Dock
Nettle
Dry Beet Powder
Dried Watercress
Parsley
Dandelion Root
Dulse

Calcium Tea: 1 part chamomile
1 part comfrey
1 part borage
1 part oat straw

Steep 35 - 40 minutes.

These two teas are recipes much akin to "stews". Everyone has their family favorite. Here are two of mine: Teas to help absorb minerals, so vital for menstrual well-being.

To aid elimination during menstruation, drink a tea of the following:

Equal parts:　Yellow Dock Root　　　　Nettles
Red Clover Blossoms　　and
Burdock Root　　　　　　Cassia Bark (Chinese cinnamon)

Mexican Tea (Chenopodium ambrosoides L.) To reduce profuse menses and to relieve post-delivery pains (after-birth or involution).

Painted Cup (Castilleja linariaefolia), also known as Indian paintbrush. Hopi used to aid against excessive menstrual discharge. In their language, this plant is also known as pola Mansi "Red Flower". A decoction of the pola Mansi was used to dry up the menstrual flow.

Another formula from Elaine Muhr for the alchemists in the audience: *

FEMALE REGULATOR NO. 3 for profuse menstruation. No. 198	Drachms
1. Colic Root - Gives tone and energy to the uterus.	6
2. Beth Root - Strengthens the female reproductive organs.	6
3. Geranium Root - Powerful astringent; arrests bleeding.	4
4. Squaw Root - Stimulates normal contraction of the uterus.	6
5. Erigeron - Arrests hemorrhages, contracts tissues.	4
6. Shepherds Purse - Promotes contraction of blood vessels , stops bleeding.	4

Pennyroyal oil if placed on your forehead in the spot called your third eye will result in "cramps", or uterine contractions and may help you to release the endometrium. Or take an herbal sauna to help you relax and let the flow begin. A few drops of the herbs infused in oil (cold-pressed vegetable or seed oils) like pennyroyal oil put in a pan of water on the hot rocks or stove in your sauna will let your skin "drink" the essences - or the fresh herbs will do the same placed in the heated water or hung up around the sauna.

While we're at menstruation, there are many teas to help relax you, thus making your flow a pleasureable (yes, pleasureable!) experience. Chamomile, valerian, red raspberry leaves are the best known and most readily available. Periwinkle and motherwort will relieve congestion. **For cramps ,** menstrual yoga.
        THE FOLLOWING RECIPES are recommended:

Equal parts: Yarrow   Equal parts: Mugwort
               Mint   Cramp Bark
               Elderflowers   Oat Straw
                                                        Chamomile

Foot baths of **any** of the above are often a great relief as are whole body baths with your herbal tea strained right-into the bath water. Your pores drink in the essences to soothe **you, also.**

I find that fasting on herbal teas the first day or so of bleeding is helpful (See diet section of this chapter.). Also watermelon (Take alone at a meal without other foods.) and bananas adjust hormones also.

A Formula No. 195, published by Elaine Muhr is as follows for painful and spasmodic menstruation: "The Female Regulator Tea No. 2"

---

* **Herbs**, by Elaine Muhr, 1974, P. 93. To prepare properly, steep one dose in two cups of boiling water, taking one cup morning and evening.

1. *Papoose Root - Indian remedy to facilitate menstruation.*   4
2. *Cypripedium Root - Stimulates the nervous system.*   4
3. *Cramp Bark (Viburnum Opulus) - Relaxes spasma, relieves cramps.*   8
4. *Life Root Herb - Promotes menstrual flow.*   6
5. *Blue Skullcap - Quiets the nerves, relieves cramps.*   4
6. **Figwort - Relieves pain in difficult menstruation.**   4

Mix well and divide into 20 doses, using herbs especially cut for tea.

*For profuse menstruation, look to diet and amount of toxins taken into one from the environment. (The image Kali may help here.) Dead-nettle, white or blend (Lamium album. L.). See Laura Burns' article in **Well Being** "To Help Your Flow" for more formulas for menstruation, to aid elimination, strengthen your system, and normalize it. William LeSassier's first article on Herbal Birth Control has an excellent recipe for re-storing estrogen balance and "Getting off the Pill", again by Laura, is highly recommended. All stress the wholistic approach to healing oneself by using them with respect.*

*More on pain in menstruation: If **immediately before** the menstrual flow, it's often indicative of uterine flexion meaning that the position of the womb is abnormal. Uterine flexion often occurs in women who are very thin and have lost the internal fat and the ligament upon which the uterus is suspended has lost tone. Inclined boards, as well as a carefully designed exercise program are helpful, and so are diet modifications. If pain **precedes** the period, this usually shows that there's ovarian dysfunction. This is a glandular indication that diet needs looking into. Hot Sitz baths for local treatment on alternate nights before the menstruation is due, for a week before, is soothing and helps bring about a cure.[6] If pain is **at the time of ovulation**, in either side of the abdomen, sometimes following the utero-scaral ligament around the back, it is called **mettlschmerz** meaning "middle pain" in German. This is a valuable sensation because it lets you know that you're fertile. If you do not want to be pregnant, yet are fertile, a pain sometimes manifests as a signal. When the pain **is during** the menstrual flow, it usually means the womb is inflamed itself. An inflamed womb is an acutely pelvic drama in need of immediate healing.*

*In the **Natural Way to Sexual Health**, Dr. Bieler diagnoses a woman's health by the quality of the menstrual blood. If cramping severely, he suggests it is because of the irritation to the uterus by a highly toxic discharge going through. The blood at menstruation is indicative of either the inadequate digestion of (1) starches and sugars (profuse **bright red** blood accompanied by uterine cramps) or (2) of protein rotted and putrefied (**dark** blood which is stringy, smelly - due largely to meat, eggs and cheese).*

*Now a Zuni woman, oblivious to laboratories, would spread heated sand on the floor of her home in a thick mound. She **then** sits over the sand catching her robes up around her waist. The veil, the cape - a blanket falls loosely from her shoulders to the ground. The sand, as well as her body, are covered and enclosed.*

Drachma = dram = 1/16 oz.

A woman who bleeds "too long" i.e. becomes anemic every menstruation may examine her diet and care of her physical/emotional/subtle bodies in general. A Cheyenne squaw would powder the stems and flowers of a local herb called Erigonum subalpinum. A tablespoon made a strong tea that acted at once. Perhaps herbs are also true healers in that they treat the causes and not just the symptoms. It seems that in the disagreement of eminently qualified nutritionists about the value of "mucusless" diets, macrobiotic, sproutarian, vegetarian, breathtarian, etc., herbs come out unscathed. All seem to credit the nutritive as well as medicinal value for menstrual cycles. For this reason I focus now on how herbs can help women understand their own bodies - through health, through awareness.

With awareness, we explore "changes" our bodies/psyches experience. Menstruation must be explored completely by every fertile woman, in her own way, and at her own pace.

1. *I often know menstruation is about to begin when I get an urge to clean our house. Or get into forgotten closets and reorganize them. Drawers and tubs of water also are fascinating. These are thought as symbolic for the process of emptying that occurs through menstruation.*

2. *The pleasure of living can be only as full as I allow. Holding back tears or blood/fluid at menses holds back my joy. The two don't necessarily **have** to come together. Please regard these sharings as my confession and not feel you need do it the **same** way. I know how good formulas and guarantees feel . . . yet each of us will express our own menstrual rituals, as unique as we all are.*

3. *Mom was also attuned to the deeper understandings of sexuality and fertility. As a toddler, I remember asking her "where do babies **really** come from?". In this way I wondered aloud with her how God knew when a couple were married and then it was O.K. to get pregnant. She then explained the facts-of-life – literally, enthusiastic only to the point of being inspiring and truthful. She added, God gives a woman and a man a baby when their love is just too much for **TWO**.*

4. *Menstruation was no big deal. My sister and I both knew when mom was bleeding and we were especially sensitive to the power of her feelings at that time.*

5. *This last period, I'd scheduled two astrology readings and kept my committment to them. During that time, I hardly dropped any blood. Four hours later, when I could focus on myself all alone, the flow picked up and made up for the lost time. I was reminded my experiences in birthings when women would stop their labor (dilation) - medically termed "uterine inertia" when focusing outwards. Perhaps someone came into their space with whom there was unfinished, contractual business. Then labor picks up and gets heavy a bit later when the tense situation is resolved. In any case, I believe uteruses sometimes might stop functioning so as to birth the baby at an astrologically auspicious time. Perhaps the baby wants to be gemini rising and retards the labor. Who knows? But (for example) using drugs (pitocin or other synthetic oxytocics) to "speed up" a labor is most often pitiful. Even using herbs, too, is tampering in God's plan. Consider carefully your impatience before administering to a laboring woman any remedy. And be clear just **who** is playing God. See "Placenta Recipes" for more insights on birthing.*

6. *Since I reported this in the summer of 1977, my very next period was a wowzer! Three days of deep flowing. Very pleasurable, but lots of blood! Never one to categorize myself, anyway.*

7. *I'm suspicious about laboratory work for "objective" reportings about sex. The findings are valid for the participants of the experiments only and really shouldn't be presented as some kind of procrustean bed the rest of a "normal" population should fit into when they experience sexual sharings. Always intuited that it takes a very special person to be monitored in a laboratory during sexual encounters, and that as I don't imagine myself desiring the same, all the "facts" from her experience may be very different from my own.*

8. *I've also read that tampons contain chemicals for clotting blood - with references to these as unhealthy!*

Nothing endures
unless it has first been translated
into a myth
& the great advantage of myths
is that they are ladies
with portable roots.

(- author unknown)

2

Infertility

This chapter is for those of us who are now infertile and would like to conceive. If you are interested in being sterile, either temporarily or permanently, refer to Chapter 6. A lot of the information may be regarded as "superstitious" and interesting folklore. Then again, we may read the reported rituals metaphorically; as the ways women for thousands of years have done and continue to respond to their conditions of infertility.

I had one bout with infertility for about four months a few years ago. And I'm not talking about the time of nursing - induced amenorrhea here. That space of lactation was most definitely an experience of **fertility**, though there were no monthly ovulations and menstruations. What I'm referring to here is a time in my life when I desired very much to conceive a baby, and had lots of potent sperm visiting me. My egg, **womb-nest** and as I mentioned before, desire, were also in agreement yet there were no conceptions, no baby. My mate and I valued this as a time to unhook from our images as fecund gods and godesses: this fertility queen was not getting pregnant! That realization helped loosen my hold on another fantasy - that each unprotected sexual encounter would result in a baby, one that up until now had been my only experience. The first time we didn't use our prophylactics eight years ago, we conceived Loi. Now here we were, four years later, trying to conceive our second baby. The catch here is - we put our order in for a **boy** baby. As described in **Prenatal Yoga & Natural Birth**, with the aid of astrological, tantric breath affirmation and "biological information" such as the PH alkalinity/ acidity of my cunt, position of intercourse, time of month, etc., we attempted to play God and have a boy baby. The epilog to this is that as soon as we let go of our preference in the matter and not really cared if we **had** a girl or a boy baby, we conceived **two** girl babies! This is our experience with Polly Berends' observations about infertility. She points out how couples who, believing themselves infertile, signed adoption papers and **then** become pregnant. When you give up trying to **get** pregnant, or **give** birth, and settle into **being** a parent, conception happens. Baba Hari Dass writes about people thinking of themselves as doers, so making a baby is limited by thoughts - that it's just something to **do**. Swami Satchidananda says God gives one a baby - not really the other way around. And Kahlil Gibran expressed the same idea like this - Your children will come **through** you, and not **for** you.

Infertility can be a heart-breaking problem for many of us. It is hard to imagine your sister's grief at not being able to become pregnant when by far the majority of women prefer not to conceive, and many use abortions as their birth control techniques. Yet these lists of herbs were gathered with you in mind - **doing** something about your problem helps much more than feeling sorry for yourself. Herbs are such a beautiful way to introduce you to the reality of tiny growing things - and like babies, they are deceptively powerless in appearance. But anyone who hangs out with babies, and every herbalist must agree here, that **both** are little manifestations of growing energies and are very powerful indeed!

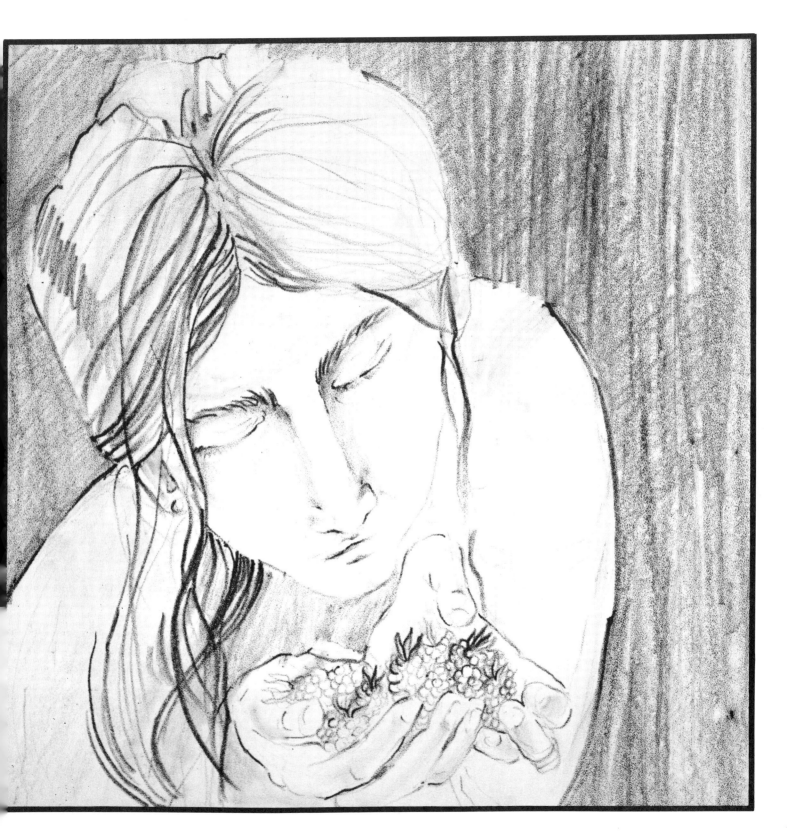

Getting off synthetic hormones is another cause for infertility and will be discussed in the chapter on Balancers and Toners. So for those of you who have just gotten off the Pill (depending on how long you took it - 'one day' to 'years' can be "just off the Pill"), please skip to that section first in Balancers and Toners.

One other way to conceive - sign adoption papers! I can't tell you how many students in my natural child-birth classes come with a small adopted child and their first pregnancy - sometimes after years of trying! Help someone else out first. You might tell a woman considering an abortion that you'll take the baby and care for her. Also, in the appendix is an article written by an astrologer on infertility. You have to be facile in the language of astrology to understand it - and that's why it's in the appendix. Her main point, however, is that sometimes in "God's plan", some of us are called upon never to be biological mothers - and this is important from the standpoint of soul-making. This is what **you as a soul** needs to understand this time around.

And now, let's look at some of the reasons for infertility on a biological level*. When there are no monthly bleedings, called amenorrhea (See chapter on Emmenagogues.) most likely there's an endocrine imbalance. The liver is very much involved here - it contributes to the regulation of the sexual hormones. Most of us ingest through food and water and air pollution many toxins - and our livers, whose job it is to de-toxify, can get very upset. That is another reason to avoid all processed, chemicalized foods - do our daily purification practices (yoga), and exercise to a full sweat - as ways to rid the body of these poisons. Raymond Dextreit recommends using clay poultices on the abdomen, over the liver, as another way to draw out toxins. See **Our Earth, Our Cure.** We now use clay often in our family for all sorts of healthful and cosmetic purposes and I highly recommend his book. Hip baths are also recommended, as well as foot-baths to increase circulation and bring a greater feeling of well-being. If you've missed your period for reasons other than pregnancy, synthetic hormone withdrawal - this recipe for glandular troubles is indicated:

Decoction - take two tablespoons of this mixture per cup of water. Bring to a boil and then simmer for two minutes. Dextreit then suggests you take 10.2 cups daily, in between meals:

Buckthorn	30 gr.	Absinth	10 gr.
Mugwort	30 gr.	Angelica	10 gr.
Yarrow	30 gr.	Marigold	10 gr.
Catnip	20 gr.	Sweet Rush	10 gr.
Costmary	20 gr.	Wild Celery	10 gr.

We can help our younger sisters by teaching them natural birth control and guiding them away from synthetic hormones. Using these when very young often causes ovarian cysts and may lead to sterility in later life. Often hereditary influences are at work - and not just because you have the same diet as your family, either. X-radiations of mothers when carrying their female babies are implicated, as well as other medical treatments for obstetrical/gynecological disorders. How many of us have been told by a gynecologist that we have "tipped wombs"? This may be a cause for sterility - but it can be remedied by natural cures. Applying poultices of herbs and/or clay can bring a tipped uterus back in alignment with the body. But a word of caution - being told by the doctor that **our** wombs are tipped and that we may have trouble getting pregnant should be taken with a grain of salt. I know too many women that got pregnant just to prove the doctor wrong. During phases of a woman's ovulation cycle, her womb lowers and raises; in other words, changes position and this is a clue to where one is - a highly nestled womb goes along with ovulation. A womb riding low in the vaginal canal is closer to menstruation. Tipped forward is sometimes our metaphorical statement of being "upfront" with a desire for sex and/or baby-making. Uterus tipped backwards may signal our innermost desire to "back away" from sexuality, in the uterine sense. Wombs do move - that's basically what I am saying here. If you're infertile because of this, **you can also change this condition.**

Sprouted wheatgrass (See Hipprocrates Health Institute for further information), which contain large amounts of Vitamin E is very helpful in cases of infertility. Also, all other sprouts - and flower salads - dress up your **daily** salad with the blossoms of wild radish, borage, marigold, nasturtium - I know there's many others but these are my favorites. Again, **doing** something about your infertility may help beyond your wildest expectations. But in the meantime, practice being motherly to see if this is what you **really** desire. Perhaps the wish for children is coming from somewhere outside of oneself - your husband wants a baby, your family, your culture. Check it out in those silent moments - visualize yourself as pregnant, as a nursing mother, as a servant. Baba Hari Das says, "Be your children's servant". If you're not willing to take on this job 24 hours a day, be a part-time mom (I'll offer my kids). There are plenty of babies being born in need of nourishment already. Make friends with a pregnant lady and help her out - clean her house, hold her babe while she goes to the bathroom (after the birthing), and move some of your maternal love through this way. This too can be a very satisfying experience. And you get to sleep through the night time too!

Once you've established natural, healthful ways of being in your world, once you've deeply checked out just what it is you might want from becoming a mother - and once you've let go your need to get pregnant, it may happen. If not, enjoy the babies already here and the ability to make love anytime, any place without the fear of pregnancy. This too can be a gift.

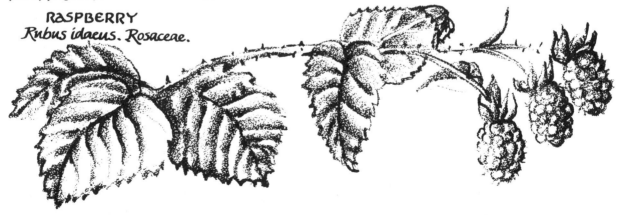

RASPBERRY
Rubus idaeus. Rosaceae.

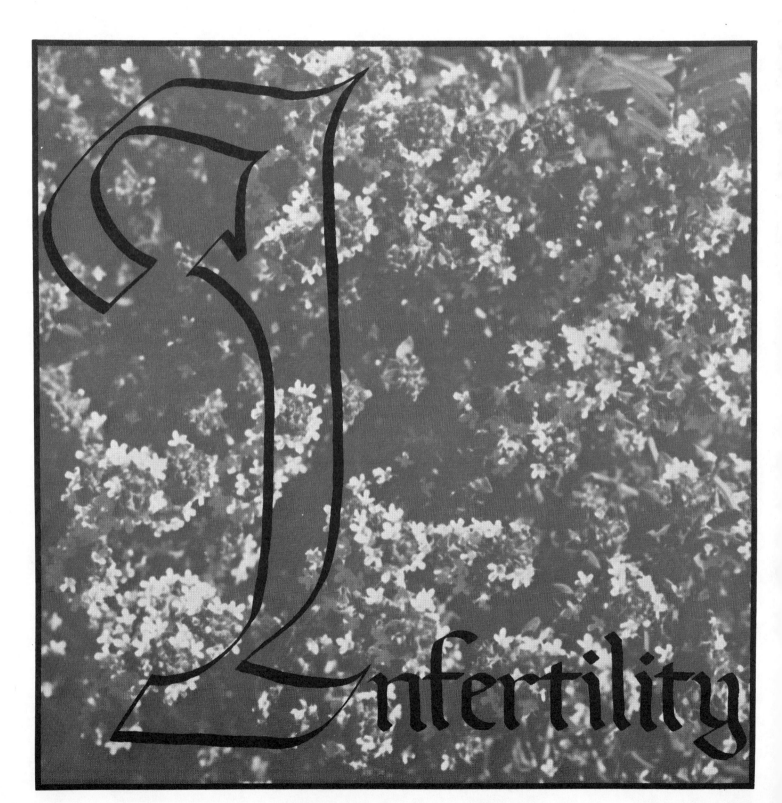

Infertility

Infertility

Balm   *Melissa officinales. Labiatae. "Beloved By Bees", "Garden Balm", "Sweet Balm", "Lemon Balm". She is a well-known monastery fragrance and used by nuns and monks for healing salves. She safeguards against early senility and impotency, says the medieval herbalist, Paracelsus. She aides prevention of infertility, and painful or delayed menses. Also facilitates release of afterbirth. For all uterine disorders. Enjoy her raw in salads. Fragrance of lemons. Good as an herbal bath to rid one's self of melancholy. Relieves nausea, vomiting, hysteria, and sexually irritating conditions. Increases menstrual flow. A member of the mint family.*

Take 2 - 4 grams of the leaves or entire plant by scalding the leaves with a cup of boiling water. Never allow the tea to boil.

*Jethro Kloss lists this fine herb as one of the **best** herbs for curing general female troubles.*

Melissa or Balm   *Used by Arabian physicians for "affections of the heart". According to Paracelsus, balm was a rejuvenator, if steeped in wine, an important ingredient of love potions.*

Blue Skullcap   *Scutellaria galericulata. Labiatae. "Mad-dog Weed", "Skull cap", "Hooded Willow Herb". A cure for sterility when used internally as a brew of the whole plant, taken in a wineglass, full, morning and night, or externally as a lotion or douche. Very quieting, a nervine with catnip and hops. "Splendid to suppress unwanted sexual desire", as stated by Kloss. Useful for helping morphine addicts "kick".*

Cayenne   *"Capsicum" from Cayenne, South America - "the biting herb", KAPTO means "I bite" in Greek. Many varieties from all over Africa, West Indies, Americas, etc. When combined with bayberry, makes an unfailing remedy to check profuse menstrual bleeding. Just a smidgen - very heating herb! A little sprinkled on socks on cold days will prove very warming indeed. It has been rumored that vultures avoid carcasses that have ingested quantities of "the biting herb".*

Clover   *See Red Clover.*

Lady's Mantle   *Alchemilla vulgaris. Rosaceae. "Alkemelich", the arabic name meaning alchemist, the ancestors of chemists. For treating infertility and restoring normal menstruation, curing excessive flow. A specific for women's ailments; a tonic for the organs of generation and the Arabs claim, if taken from one period to another, the woman will **conceive** Also a heart tonic. Culpepper says "Helps with over-flagging breasts". The history of this magic herb goes on. The leaves have the property of secreting water droplets in the morning . . . These*

42

silver droplets collect on tiny hairs on the surface of the leaf. Alchemists used to gather the drops (like Bach flower remedies), as they thought that this heavenly water would aid them in preparing the philosopher's stone. Also a real help in childbirth. Promotes healing of wounds and staunching of blood after birthing.

Scald the whole plant in one cup water.

Licorice Root (wild)

Glycyrrhiza lepidota. Nutt. A root decoction has been used to induce menstruation. Part of Le Sassier's hormonal balancing formula, very important for those desiring conception. Contains estrogenic substances. Delicious! Chewed on, said to make you passionate or at least help to awake sexual energy. Also used to hasten delivery of the placenta or when the mother had after fever. Glycyrrhiza glabralieguminosae: used for treating infertility. Glychrrhiza glabra: was stored in large amounts in King Tut's tomb to aid in soul's journey (a nice metaphor for reincarnation). Licorice was a cure-all in Eygptian times and highly regarded by the Chinese herbalists for thousands of years. Included in Dr. Christopher's "Change-Ease" formula. Also called amolillo and used for cleansing the uterus after birth.

Take the whole fresh plant, crush it and cook in a quart of slowing, rolling, boiling water. Drink with meals unstrained.

Mandrake

Mandragora officinarum. "Mandragora", "Barass". A mystified herb, an herb with "sexual connotations - used by Jews in olden times to cast out demons, probably because of the root's resemblance to an androgynous human body. The value of mandrake as an aid to conception is found in Genesis, Chapter 30,0, being used as barter, bringing Leah and Jacob their fifth son. French herbalists call mandrake the herb of beaten women due to the berries' and bark's healing properties for bruises. Arabian herbalists call mandrake the devil's apple and French say it's the love-apple; a name given also to the juicy, red member of the nightshade family, tomatoes. In Pliny's time, a gathering ceremony was of standing with one's back to the wind, drawing 3 circles around the plant with a sword, pouring a libation and then turning to the west in order to uproot the mandrake. Such traditions on the gathering of the mandrake plant have imbued some mystery about this herb. Used in love potions to facilitate pregnancy, and correct female infertility, mandragora is also connected with devil legends. Josephus, Jewish writer, first described the sound of the shreiking mandrake when it is uprooted. Mandrake was used by witches to increase clairvoyance. American Indians used Podophyllum pelatum or American mandrake for uterine diseases and knew it as a de-obstructant. Also used by the Indians for magical purposes. Also known as "mayapple" or "racoon-berry". True mandrake is in short supply and white byrony is often substituted for it, since the 16th century and on, when mandrake was selling for $57.50 - $69.00 for one root. Truly an herb to be used respectfully. **Boiled it is lethal!!** But as my friend Rab Madrone Menzies says, more people have been killed by people than by wild plants!

Marijuana

Cannabis sativa. See "Herbs for the Mind".

Orchis   *Orchis masculata or Chidaceae. The root tubers are the most important part of this herb. Best sun dried and crushed. The powder is used in Arabia as Sahleb and in Turkey as Saleo. Made into a drink with warmed milk and given to infants being weaned, to restore sexual vigor in women and men, and for those who are infertile.*

Take 2 oz. of Salep powder to 3/4 pint hot water. Mix with equal amount of warm milk; flavor with cinnamon. Drink one cup morning and night. May give for difficult labor, but without the milk. Aphrodisiac, and also used for abortion and anemia.

Raspberry Leaf   *Rubus idaeus. Rosaceae. The pregnant woman's best herbal friend. But raspberry is also used as reproductive organ toner. The foliage of this plant contains **fragrine**, which has a special effect on the female organs. The muscles of the pelvic region, as well as the muscles in the womb, will be tonified by daily drinking of this herb. Also used to bring out the placenta. Kloss reports it decreases the menstrual flow. It relieves morning sickness and is an aid to an easy birthing. Juliette de Baircli Levy writes that it's rare for a Gypsy woman to go thru pregnancy without drinking daily raspberry from time of conception and gives birth with the ease of the "wild vixen".*

If needy of a strong dose to deliver placenta, give every 2 or 3 hours concentrated raspberry tea with a tsp. of crushed Ivy leaves to every 2 tsp. of Raspberry. It is also helpful against sterility and prized for helping infertile women and men to conceive.

Red Clover   *Trifolium pratense. Leguminosae. Considered by herbalists to be a "God given remedy". de Baircli Levy. Much valued for her alkaline quality restoring fertility and relieving leukorrhea. Used to purify the blood and though this hasn't been my focus for this book on herbs, healthy "alkaline" blood is vital for women's general health. The chlorophyll is especially important for this. Ann Wigmore writes on this subject in great and glorious detail. See bibliography.*

Red Raspberry   *See Raspberry.*

Red Sage   *See Sage.*

Skullcap or Scullcap   *Scutellaria lateriflora. "Helmet flower", "Blue pimpernel", "Hoodwort", "Mad weed". Very soothing to excitable nerves. "Splendid to suppress undue sexual desire". - Kloss.*

Scutellaria galericulata. Labiatae. Known as a treatment for sterility and used internally (douche) or externally (lotion) - Levy. Riva writes that if a wife wears scullcap, it insures her husband from being seduced by others.

Summer Savory   *Satureja hortensis. Taken warm as a remedy for suppressed menses. Increase the menstrual flow. You probably best know this herb in the kitchen. Used widely with marjoram. Has been reported to be an herb used in treating infertility.*

Watercress   *Nasturtium officinale. Cruoferae. "Scurvy grass". Eat in salads and enjoy a taste addition of much manganese and other organic minerals without the oxalic acid. Very high in Vitamins E and C. Used in treatment of scanty or failing milk supply. Good for treating uterine cysts. The old name for watercress was the "poor man's bread". ZINC, an essential mineral for healthy reproductive functioning, will help birth control users recover from those synthetic cycles. Needed for proper pituitary functioning. Get it from seeds, nuts, green veggies, mushrooms, onions and even maple syrup. Zinc is lost if you throw out cooking water, eat diuretics or foods which contain nitrates or nitrites. (Formerly called saltpeter and used to dampen sexual desire by destroying zinc in system. Saltpeter is also used in fireworks.) Read those processed foods' labels! If you can't pronounce it, don't eat it. Parvati's golden rule of nutrition.*

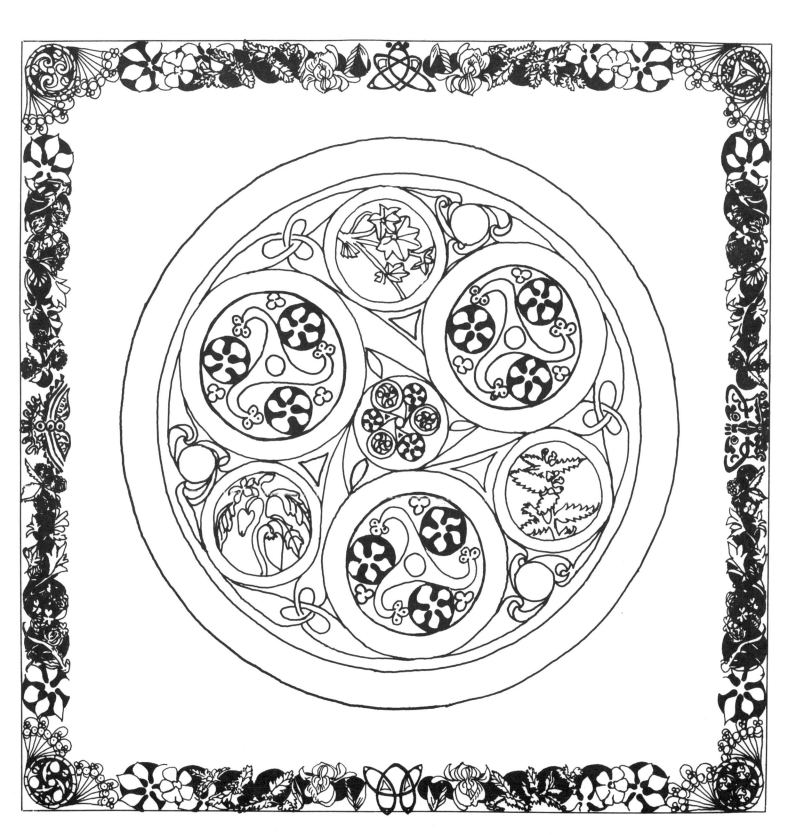

August 6, 1976

Dear Jeannine,

I have a copy of your Pre-natal Yoga Book and enjoy it. I have never been pregnant but I look forward to it with anticipation. Ever since I knew what being pregnant was, I've dreamed of being in that state while at the same time hoping and trying not to become pregnant! Quite a paradox, eh!

I started my birth control history by taking the pill at 17. Off and on over a 2 year period I took it a total of 8 months. Every time I went on it out of convenience and every time I quit out of disgust. My attitudes about sex were a little strange while taking it. I hated taking pills so much that I felt everyday I took one had to be justified by an act of sex. That leads to a lot of weird pressures, etc. So off the pill I went for the last time, swore I'd never, ever go back on it.

After the pill came the diaphram. I liked it a lot. A little messy but easy to use and no drugs, etc. Stopped using it in April of this year because we were living in a very un-private situation and I found it hard to use in a public situation!

On to the I.U.D.! This is on a par with the pill for grotesqueness. I'm now in the process of having mine removed after 4 months of use. I hate the thought of having it inside of me. Have had a few problems with it, bleeding, cramps, etc. Had the I.U.D. put in to try it out and see if it was the answer to all of my B.C. problems. Answer - definitely not.

So, it's back to the diaphram which I look at with fond eyes now. Am determined to make it work for me. I have never tried any method of psychic B.C. Would like to be more sure of my mind over body control before I do.

I read everything I find on Birth Control (B.C.). Am hopeful that someday I will be able to have sex without fear of an unwanted pregnancy and most important without man-made contraceptions.

Love,
Ruth

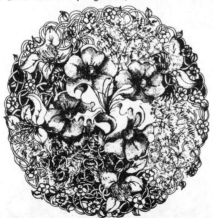

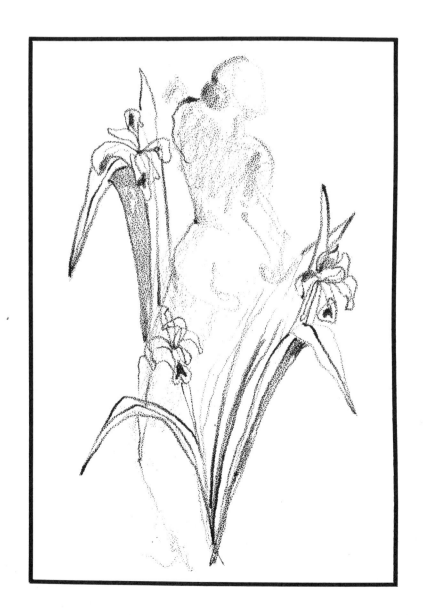

48

3

Herbal Birth Control

*The following herbs have been divided into arbitrary categories of either (1) those that cause permanent sterility and (2) those that create conditions of temporary infertility. Actually, all the herbs listed in this book are aids towards developing a form of natural[1] birth control by helping you to become in tune with yourself as a healthy, sexual being. Herbal abortives have purposefully been overlooked. I consider them dangerous. Most women do not realize that they must still **give birth** to a poisoned or dislodged fetus when undergoing an herbal abortion. I have one friend who counsels a woman through herbal abortions. She makes sure after several interviews and meditations that this is what the **woman truly needs, and then gives her a brew. The aborting woman must spend that time isolated in a teepee on her land, and my friend visits her often to help her psychically let go of the baby. The aborted fetus is then handled by the mother, to literally get in touch with all facets of an herbal abortion. This is obviously not an easy way out, yet it does circumvent to a large degree most later guilt that befalls even the stoutest woman who has the doctor "do it for her". But this is a chapter on "birth control" - a misnomer, for it sounds more like a hospital childbirth preparation class than a tool to avoid conception. Some herbs make you infertile for a little while (or longer) and others are reported to permanently make you sterile. I personally feel that my cycles of fertility are given to be understood and to be played within - not something to irretrievably cut away, or remedy through the use of herbs. But then again, another baby would not be considered a "mistake" in a method, a failure to be erased. So my perspective, one might say, is priviledged. This is the reason I've included these herbs for birth control.*

HERBS HAVE BEEN USED FOR THOUSANDS OF YEARS FOR CONTRACEPTION. The earliest of birth control recipes were formulated by Sun-Semo in China during the first century A.D. One of his prescriptions indicated that the woman should "take some oil and quicksilver and fry in oil one full day. Take one pill as large as a jujube seed on an empty stomach and it will forever prevent one from becoming pregnant . . . it will not injure the person". An earlier Indian remedy was "One tola (about half an ounce) of powdered palm leaf and red chalk taken with cold water on the fourth day of menstruation makes a woman sterile with certainty". Soranos, a Greek (98-139 A.D.), invented the following: "Pine bark, rhus, coriaria, both to equal parts: pulverize it with wine shortly before coitus with the help of wool". Though this isn't an herbal contraceptive, I can't resist reporting it. From the Middle Ages, Alfred the Great, an alchemist, seriously recommended this: "If a woman spit thrice in the mouth of a frog, or eat bees,[2] she will not become pregnant." Now all I need to find is a yawning frog. He also suggested soaking a piece of cloth in barberry oil and placing it on a woman's temples for contraception. From Ezekial 47:12 to the present, in adoration for the power of herbs, womankind has often used these plants of compassion towards greater well-being.

Before diving into the wealth of information about herbs and birth control, the noble savage myth needs

Fertility Control Recipe, 1550 B.C.
The Ebers Papyrus, a compendium of medical writings dating at the latest from 1550 B.C., contains this prescription, probably the first for a contraceptive—a medicated lint tampon designed to "cause that a woman should cease to conceive for one, two, or three years."

*a new look. A common archetype now floating around is the "natural woman", probably living in a non-technological society, who is steeped in the flora of her living space - very close to the earth. When talking about childbirth, it is **she** who births the baby painlessly and almost nonchalantly, alone out in the woods, and then resumes in a matter of minutes her usual daily tasks (and none the worse for wear). Her mythic sister in the natural birth control arena can use those plants that grow around her in order to control conceptions (or abort "mistakes") without any side effects. Of course, supportive culture via daily rituals and sharings of plant lore are a part of this phenomenon. Now I believe this is the hope of many women (and men) returning to their natural cycles. What I'd like to include here is the reality of our heroines, the "primitive women of other cultures", and their very frequent practice of infanticide. Killing unwanted infants is a widespread population control technique[1] and this shouldn't be overlooked.*

The preceding investigation into abortion and infanticide helped me detach from the noble savage ideal quite quickly. And, more importantly, it let me see through my desire to have that magical plant which would make me infertile at will for a time span of my choice. This desire, to be at one with nature and simultaneously in control of nature, is the main force feeding all my energy behind "herbal birth control". The following is an account of a native American woman's attempts to understand the relationship between plants and fertility. It is a personal account of how ancestors continue to live through us. In this case, the American Indians and their relationship to the Earth and her children called herbs.

THE FOLLOWING ARE THE WORDS OF A NATIVE AMERICAN WOMAN AND HER HERBAL BIRTH CONTROL EXPERIENCE:

"In search for my roots and in search for myself, I see in my 'progressive' society the capacity to drive anything natural toward extinction. Webster defines natural as something being produced or existing in nature: something not artificial or manufactured. The television media is introducing bionic people. Human robots: a new and improved human being. They can outrun, outjump, and out do old regular people any day. The population is becoming more and more dependent on cities. The trend has been shifting away from any type of naturalness. It's frightening. I don't agree with many of the modes of my society, but what else is there? What are some alternatives? In answer to my questions, I look toward my ancestors, Native Americans. A people with natural practices. In this paper, I look at their ways and how they traditionally deal with the natural functions of the woman's life cycle. I will present the opinion of Native American Indians on the subjects of menstruation, and birth control .

I'm searching for alternatives because trends of modern society scare me. I look around and see additives in food that are to enhance the taste of my food and chemicals that are added to extend the life of the food. To relieve the cramps due to my monthly flow of blood, my society recommends a little blue pill. This blue pill called Midol will alleviate those awful discomforts .

I see contradictions in this society, I'm told to strive for independence, but then I'm to conform and rely on someone for medical help. I'm told to depend on the doctor to deliver my child. Why con't I do it myself? Why am I not capable? They say the best way is their way, nice and sterilized. Sterilized means free from germs, free from emotions. It sounds like a vacuum: no warmth of love .

"When I look for ways to practice contraception, I have many choices. There is a pill that will alter my metabolism and regulate my menstruation. It works, they say. I see how it works too: I see how it can cause me great pain or kill me, eventually, through cancer .

"Another choice is the intra-uterine device, or I.U.D. A very modern convenience, I'm sure. Its function is not to prevent conception, as with the pill[3], but to induce abortion if conception occurs.

*My intention here to focus on the four categories named above, beginning with the most serious one first: herbs that cause permanent sterility. For those of us very firm in our decisions not to bear children, medical technology offers us several forms of relief. These are mixed blessings, as are all technological tools. Some women who choose hysterectomies as foolproof birth control have ended up proving how foolish this can be **as a solution**; tubal pregnancies have been reported to occur anyway so the women must then again have more surgery to remove their tubes. Tubal ligations or any form that interrupts the descent of the egg is grossly blocking "letting go" and outward energy flow. I am of the belief that all disease can be traced to interferences of natural energy flows. The wound of affliction opens up a series of symbolic, cultural, and mythic paths of insight. Each time metal is introduced beneath the skin surface in a violent manner (requiring anesthesia to control pain) the natural energy flow is unbalanced. This is the reason that I'm including a report of herbs used for permanent sterility, as it feels like the lesser of the many evils. Coming from a philosophic space, "ridding" oneself of the "problem" of unwanted fertility is missing the point. We **choose** to be cyclically fertile beings to get in touch with some very important realizations about sexuality and responsibility. Giving away this chase after soul (psyche) each month to the surgeon's knife (or even herbal remedy) is setting oneself up for "getting it" on another level, another besides just sexually "getting it" WITHOUT having to worry anymore about pregnancy.[4] Soon enough we will step off this hormonal roller coaster becoming menopausally "liberated" and able to "get some" any time without pregnancy considerations. In the meantime, enjoy the ups and downs of being fertile and infertile, desirous and satisfied.*

"The Lakota was a true naturist; a lover of nature. He loved the earth and all things of the earth, the attachment growing with age. The old people came literally to love the soil and they sat or reclined on the ground with a feeling of being close to a mothering power. It was good for the skin to touch the earth and the old people liked to remove their moccasins and walk with bare feet on the sacred earth. Their tipis were built upon the earth and their altars were made of earth. The birds that flew in the air came to rest upon the earth and it was the final abiding place of all things that lived and grew. The soil was soothing, strengthening, healing, and cleansing .

"That is why the old Indian still sits upon the earth instead of propping himself up and away from its life-giving forces. For him, to sit or lie upon the ground is to be able to think more deeply and to feel more keenly; he can see more clearly into the mysteries of life and come closer in kinship to other lives about him .

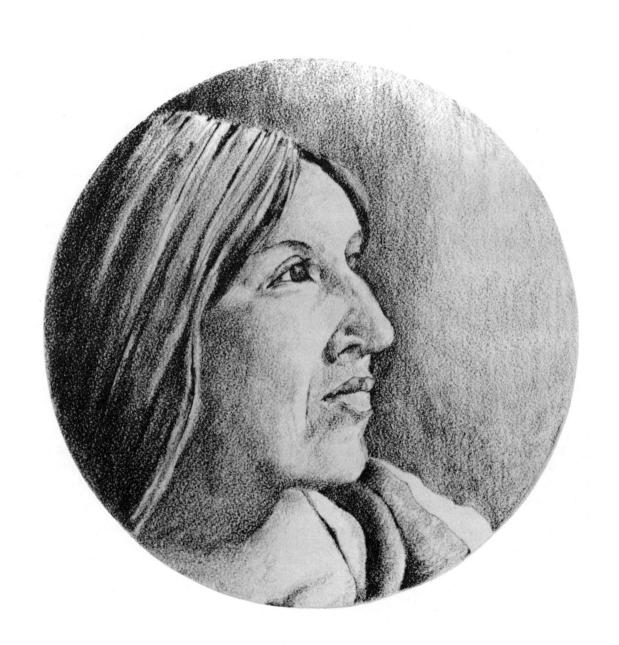

"Kinship with all creatures of the earth, sky, and water was a real, active principle. For the animal and bird world there existed a brotherly feeling that kept the Lakota safe among them, and so close did some of the Lakotas come to their feathered and furred friends that in true brotherhood they spoke a common tongue."

"The old Lakota was wise. He knew that man's heart away from nature becomes hard; he knew that lack of respect for growing, living things soon led to lack of respect for humans too. So he kept his youth close to its softening influence."[5]

"Respect. Respect for and acknowledgement of the inherent powers of all living things is necessary. In herbal remedies, if one doesn't see and feel the powers held within the herbs, that person will find no benefit from such medicines. It depends on where one's faith is placed.

"I visited a doctor some months ago. She told me of a new type of I.U.D. on the market. "It's new; it's better", she told me. She didn't mention anything about the other types of I.U.D.'s until I questioned her. I asked her to show me something that wouldn't alter my metabolism, or cause cancer, or hurt me by imbedding itself within the walls of my uterus. I asked her to show me a way in which I could practice contraception that would be healthy. "I want something good for me!", I pleaded. She had no immediate reply but in a few minutes she responded in anger. She was outraged that I dare to question her authority, or maybe she was upset because she too saw the hazards I wasn't willing to gamble with. She wouldn't listen to my thoughts and feelings on the subject, and she scoffed at my vague, at that time, notions on herbal remedies used for contraceptions. Her ways were the only ways; that's the point she got across to me by not raising her voice too much.

"Such narrow-mindedness on the doctor's part pushed me to find some more natural means of birth control. I became aware of seminars focusing on the very topic. The women involved spoke of herbs used to regulate menstruation and the powers of some herbs to induce abortion. Not much was offered as to where the information on herbs was gathered, but I soon found books dealing with what I was grasping for."[6]

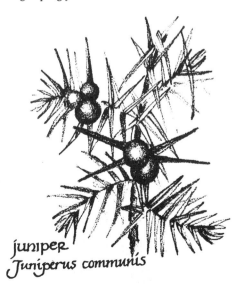

juniper
Juniperus communis

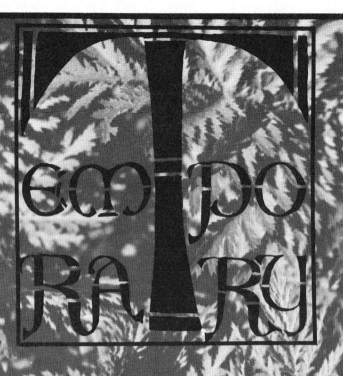

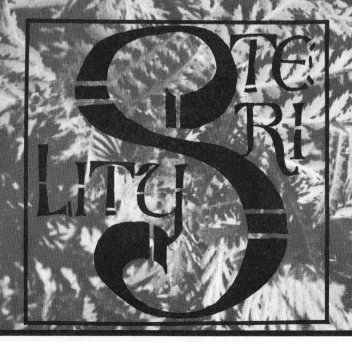

Temporary Sterility

Alum Root   *See Wild Geranium.*

Antelope Sage   *Erigonum jamesii. Navajo women boiled the root during menstruation for temporary sterility. Navajo men also reported to use this herb, along with "twisted medicine" or bahia dissecta.*

Blessed Thistle   *Onicus benedictus. "Holy thistle", "Spotted thistle". An infusion of the flower tops has been used as a contraceptive. It contains estrogen. She is a meditation herb. Women use her to produce milk. "Our Lady's Milk Thistle" root is a vegetable, the leaves a salad and the head an artichoke. It clears the mind of depression. Good for all women's discomforts. A salad of young hearts leaves and the stems stripped of their course outer coverings increases milk flow and regulate bleedings. Dr. Christopher's "Change-Ease" formula, a corrective for women's regenerative systems, includes Blessed Thistle. Good during puberty and menopause.*

Blue Cohosh   *Caulophyllum thalictroides. L. "pa". Aside from it's emmenagogic properties, "squaw root", as it's also called, can be used to stem an excessive flow. It helps to regulate one's flow. Used by Menomince, Potawatomi, and Meskwaki Indians. Cohosh is an Algonquian name which has been applied to other herbs as well. Vogel and Wiener report the Chippewas used a strong decoction as a contraceptive. For ovarian and womb. trouble, treats leukorrhea, and increases menstrual flow. Kloss.*

Deer's Tongue   *Frasera speciosa or Listris odoratissima, "Wharts tongue", "Wild vanilla" of the Pacific Coast of the U.S.A. Used in small amounts to flavor smoking mixtures. Linked with contraception, in some mysterious way and the Shoshones. A. Riva suggests dribbling the bottom of your shoes with deer's tongue and it'll tie all tongues so they cannot speak against you. She also suggests grinding thyme and deer's tongue into a fine powder, sprinkle on a sleeping person's stomach and then listen to them divulge all their secrets. You can try for three nights in a row and if still not successful, wait at least one full moon's cycle before trying again. Personally, I've found simply asking works very well.*

Desert Mallow   *Bahia disecta. Here's an example of how ritual must go with the herbal recipe. Shoshone Indians of Elko, Nevada, ensure the mother's temporary sterility by her laying in a trench of warm ashes and drinking a tea of boiled Desert Mallow and Wild Geranium. One year of infertility results.*

Dogbane   *(Spreading) Apocynum and rosaemifolium. L. See Milkweed for description. Promotes temporary sterility. Roots boiled in water and drunk once weekly. Possibly toxic. Use with caution.*

False Hellebore *Veratrum callfronicum. e. Durand. A root decoction, taken daily for three weeks, prevents conception. It is drunk daily by the Indians of Beowave, Nevada. A tea of the cured root is to insure sterility for life. Very poisonous. The Greeks used the Black Hellebore as a remedy for madness. The Germans connected it with Huldah, the marriage Goddess. I included this herb only for herstorical interest - NOT recommended at all, unless you're an Indian in Beowave, Nevada - and even then know what you're doing clearly, before using Hellebore.*

See letter, page 130.

Geranium Root *See Wild Geranium. Powerful astringent. Arrests hemorrhage.*

Gromwell *Lithospermum officinale. Boraginaceae. Lithospermum ruderale, the American species, is used by Indians as an agent to prevent conception. Gabriel. The effect seems to be derived from plant hormones.*

Holy Thistle *See Blessed Thistle.*

Indian Paintbrush *Castilleja linariae folia, "painted cup". Hopi women used it to dry up the menstrual flow and prevent contraception. This may, or may not, prevent ovulation. "Pala mansi" in Hopi language meaning "red flower". Whiting.*

Indian Turnip *Arisaema triphyllum, "jack-in-the-pulpit". Two tsp. of powdered dried root in ½ glass cold water, strained, for temporary sterility. Hopi recipe. 1 tsp. of powdered in ½ glass water, strained, contraception for 1 week.*

Juniper *(Common.) Juniperus communis L. She's emmenagogic, as well as reported to produce temporary sterility if berries are made into a tea and drunk three consecutive days. Also useful for leukorrhea. Zuni used the leaves to lessen pain in childbirth. Used for yeast infections this way: Soak a handful of berries overnight, then add a quart of boiling water. Boil for ½ hour. Let cool, strain and use as a douche. You can also put it in a humidifier. Breathe deeply for lung problems. This herb is a natural fungicide. Remember, for yeast or "the itch" problems, avoid bubble baths (take herbal baths instead), tight pants and scented toilet paper. Develop cunt consciousness.*

Milkweed *Asclepias halli. See Dogbane, spreading temporary sterility. Asclepias sytiaca. "A splendid remedy for female complaints". Boiled roots tasting similar to asparagus. Kloss. A tea of the whole plant for temporary sterility used by the Indians of Quebec.*

Poverty Weed (Am) *Iva axillaris. The Cahuilla Indians use this herb for contraception. J. Rose. This same tribe would only use the poisonous poppy (eschsholtzia calfornica) if needed and then by the witchdoctors only. May be dangerous, if used incorrectly.*

Ragleaf Bahia *Used by the Navaholas for contraception. A tea of the root is boiled for 30 minutes. It is found inside the Grand Canyon on both rims and flowers from July to November in the Tusayan area of the Park. M. Wiener, **Earth Medicines, Earth Foods.***

Thistle *Quinault Indians of Washington used the whole plant, steeped, to inhibit fertilization.*

Wild Geranium *Sphaeralcea ambigua, "storkbill". Used with Desert Mallow by Shoshone women after birth to become infertile for one year. Total Mothering (See Appendix) no doubt had something to do with the effectiveness. Also known as "Alum Root", good for leukorrhea and excellent for treating profuse menstruation. In womb troubles, as a douche. A strong solution rubbed over tits will dry up milk or just over nipples to harden them.*

Wild Ginger *Aingiver officinale. Zingiberaceae. Used as a contraception, boiled slowly in small amount of water for a long time. The root is not actually "wild" but imported from China and West Africa. Good for delayed menstruation and for exhaustion following childbirth. Also helpful as a warm drink for childbirth pains, especially with honey, lemon or molasses. It will increase the menstrual flow. Chewed, it's an immediate remedy for menstrual cramps.*

Wild Yam *Dioscorea villosa. "Colic root", "China root", "Devil's bones". The root of the Wild Yam in Mexico and Central America, contains the starting materials for the synthesis of the complex steroids which eventually go into the making the "Pill". It was also used by the Meskwakol and Chippewa Indians as a decoction to relieve labor pains.*

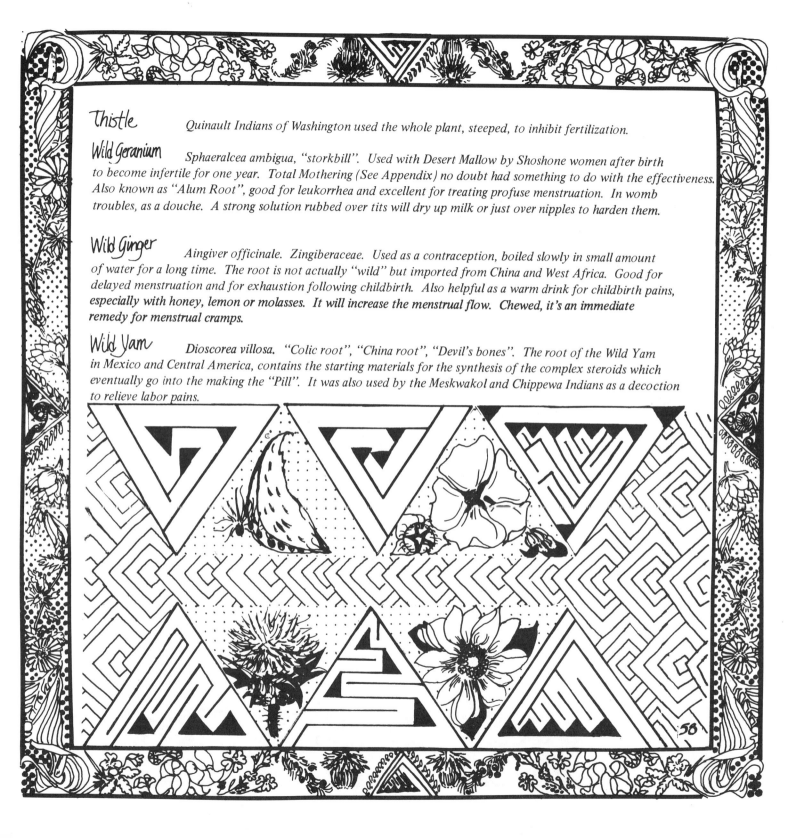

58

PERMANENT STERILITY

Permanent Sterility

False Hellebore   *Veratrum californicy e. Durand. See "Temporary Sterility".*

False Solomon's Seal   *Smilacina astellata. Nevada Indians used a root infusion to regulate menstrual disorders. See appendix for cautionary advice about this herb.*

Solomon's Seal   *Convallaria polygonatum. Excellent for all female troubles "Solomon plume". Smelacena amplexcaulis nutt. As for permanent sterility, a tea of leaves daily for one week.*

Indian Turnip   *Asarum Canadense L. See "Temporary Sterility".*

Piri Piri   *The Indians of Equador use these roots in some unknown way. J. Rose.*

Spotted Cowbane   *Circuta maculata. Cherokees would chew on the root for four days, and if it didn't kill them, they'd be forever infertile. This was considered a crime. Very dangerous.*

Stoneseed   *Lithospermum ruderale. Take the dried root, chip one handful of it, cover in water and bring to a boil. Or make a cold infusion of the chipped root. Drink daily for six months. Shoshone recipe. Use only with supervision, if at all. Very dangerous.*

*S*omewhat macrobiotically influenced, my feeling is that herbs used by women in specific geographic and cultural locations for permanent sterility **work because there is a shared and genetically coded receptivity to that end. In other words, a mutual belief system sustains the efficiency of the herbal remedy for those women.** Ritual, as well as body chemistry and diet, is important here. Perhaps that is why the Chinese herbal advertised as an amazingly long term birth control herb has been causing severe side effects in some California women.[7] Chinese herbs may be primarily **Chinese** women, i.e. for whomever recognized these plants of compassion as fellow country women and is in native resonance with them.

My hunch is population control through herbs can't be massive like the technology behind the most often-bought contraceptives. Herbs can bring back a sense of the individual's own power in sexuality and "natural family planning" and is a non-sexist form of birth control. Men can take herbs also and be involved in the relationships between plants and fertility.

But we have another need in regards to our sexual well-being. Jean Rostand wrote, "Woman pays her blood each month for failing to conceive". How many women do you know who would agree with this statement? We need to come to some truths about our responsibility to conscious conception. Using herbs as a tool into one's Self finely hones awareness - watching, handling, smelling, drinking, bathing in herbs also nourishes a sensitivity to natural forces. By using herbs we come to touch upon the world of devas and spirits who feed upon the same energies as sexual forces do. The image of finding a baby beneath a cabbage leaf illustrates the connection. Herbs can bridge the mythology. Ibn Sina, a very famous Muslim scientist, wrote a medical encyclopedia which included many contraceptive techniques, among which was the following: The woman should insert in her vagina, before and after intercourse the flowers and seeds of the cabbage plant[8], meant to be effective after dipped in a special juice (unnamed). Roasted walnuts placed inside women's clothing to become barren is used in Europe to this day. The African tribes heat up the testicles of husbands to kill sperm - roasted walnuts, eh? And over 5,000 years ago women were swallowing fried quicksilver for contraception, and if that didn't work, they'd swallow 14 tadpoles three days after menstruation. Prostitutes, who ingest large quantities of seminal fluid, are less fertile due to prostaglandin, a substance in the ejaculatory fluid. Tadpoles, eh? This is using herbs "metaphorically" for birth control.

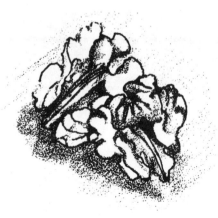

Dear Jeannine,

My attitudes are considered to be quite 'eccentric' among my friends - but I hope this helps you out with your book because I'm sure **somebody** must be interested in my experience, etc. I'm not too good at writing down my thoughts - but here goes ...

As in everything else, I think birth control is a problem only in that we make it one. I don't mean to say that it is a problem of little importance though, because while we're concerned with a 'problem', it remains one.

For myself, being almost thirty, I have a mere ten or eleven year history of dealing with the 'problem' of birth control. And my experiences with doctors, conventional methods, etc. are no where near as horrific as some women I've talked to, but certainly full of encounters with rigid, moralistic, and in too many cases, ignorant 'western M.D.'s'. I've had two abortions of which I am neither ashamed nor proud, one illegal, one legal, the latter only a little less painful, without the 'moral' overtones of the first. One thing women, and certainly men, must face is that abortion is painful emotionally no matter what, and to deny that is to suppress normal and healthy emotion. To me the suffering I went thru was a part of my decision to abort the life within me and I certainly feel I'm better off now, a few years later, for having accepted the responsibility for my actions then. There are few things that make me angrier or more frustrated tho than a so-called 'spiritual' person (particularly a male) condemning abortion as a wholly amoral, unnecessary act - because, really, who is going to suffer the brunt of that kind of thinking? Most likely, I'd say, the women involved, rarely the men involved, and how can that be justified?

I started taking the pill when I was nineteen and took them on and off 'til I was twenty eight, intermittantly using foam or rhythm or just pulling out when I'd get fed up with the effects the pill was having on my body and psyche. As a matter of fact, through the years as I became more disillusioned with our system of medicine and took to using herbal and other natural remedies in general, the area of our own womanhood is the last insecurity we let go of. Even when I wouldn't dream of going to a regular M.D. for an illness, I made my regular visit for gynecological checkup and pills. Then finally, after having been in love with and making love with the same man for 2½ years, and being aware of what the pill was doing to me, I gave it up for good. I can see now how taking pills, or using any other birth control 'method' puts the act of physical lovemaking into a separate realm in our minds - it divides our psyche, or is the symptom of a divided psyche, and sex can't be accepted as just another part of the flow of life. I'm not condemning conventional birth control methods, there is obviously a need for them, for as long as an individual feels the need for them. I do think there's a better way when we're ready for it, when we're ready to take responsibility for and control of our own lives.

I tried a copper I.U.D. for a few months, which seemingly was working well, but a doctor I went to for a checkup arbitrarily pulled it out without consulting me first. It had been the most pleasant birth control method I'd used up 'til then, so I was furious with him at the time. Now I'm grateful to him because it was the last straw for me, the last time I was going to subject myself to such disrespectful treatment. I could go on and on about how doctors have put me down for being a sexual person, caused unnecessary physical and emotional pain and demonstrated their scorn and/or indifference towards womanhood in general - even women doctors sometimes!

I did make the break then - no more doctors, no more artificial birth control methods because I'd come to fear them much more than I feared giving birth. I got a copy of a natural birth control book, which tells you how to calculate your astrological cycle and went by that for a while - but not for long. I read an article in which a woman said that she had evidence that the method worked only if the women using it believed in it - and I realized that I didn't even know if I believed in it or not. I also think that believing in what you're doing is of prime importance in how effective you are. And I really started seeing how all those birth control methods through the years were getting in the way of my sexuality, of my healthy sense of womanhood. As I began to rely on my own body's wisdom, perhaps that's called psychic birth control, I began experiencing myself as woman for the first time. This was around the time I had taken 'womancraft' too, a psychic training course to increase your positive feelings about being a woman. Although I felt some of the women involved in the class were rejecting men a bit too heavily, it was a good experience for me. Not only has lovemaking been more spontaneous and natural, but I no longer consider the fact that I'm a very sensual person as a problem. It's no longer 'how can I control it' but revelling in the multitudinous ways I can express it. I also live with a man who is sensitive, loving and supports me wholeheartedly in what I am. Childbirth is still a bit frightening to me - I did have bad conditioning in that respect - but much less so than before.

That is, of course, a very personal subjective account. I'm not advocating that everyone should throw away their pills or whatever and 'think positive'. But I do think that the time was ripe for me a year ago to place all my faith in my body and my psyche - and I think that it's also a universal experience, that a person reaches a decision like mine when they're ready. I no longer see birth control as a problem. I can't imagine now having a baby at a 'bad' time. Yet I feel that now probably isn't the best time for me and am confident I won't get pregnant. Of course only time will tell - it's possible that I'm fooling myself. If so, pretty effectively so far. But **I don't** feel that that's true, that I am fooling myself, and that's become what is most important to me - trusting my intuitions about how to live my life. While I'm not 'consciously' controlling the situation, I feel that some part of me does, and that I don't need that awareness at the fore of my mind anymore. I'm happier and certainly saner than ever before. I'm sure when I do have a child it will be a joyous experience.

The more natural we can be about expressing our sexuality, the better we exemplify the true beauty of women, and surely Humankind, in all areas of our lives.

Good luck with your book!

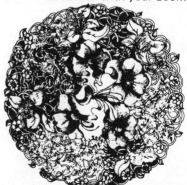

With Love,
Pat

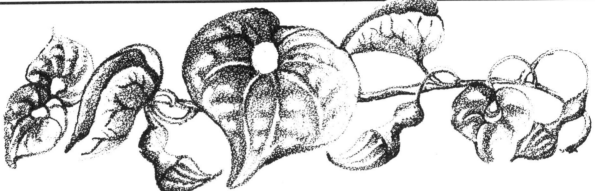

I'd like to close this chapter with the metaphor on the herb BIRTHWORT - this plant of compassion has heart-shaped leaves. Nature gently reminding us again how the heart is always involved in matters of fertility. North Africans rub themselves with the juice of this plant to make themselves immune to snake-bite (ejaculation). It heals wounds - let us let go and birth our Selves anew, naturally with herbs.

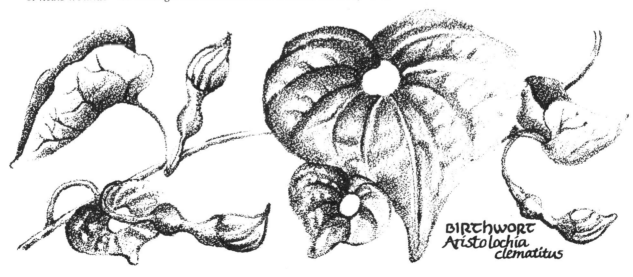

BIRTHWORT
Aristolochia
clematitus

FOOTNOTES

[1] I'm aware that the word "natural" is over-used and that all things are "chemicals", even herbs on one level.

[2] It is interesting to note that bee's pollen, contained under their wings, are his "sperm", and ingesting human sperm has been linked with reduced fertility.

[3] In reality, however, the Pill is an abortifacient also. It prevents implantation of a zygote, but doesn't necessarily intercept the union of an ovum and sperm. Webster has redefined the word "contraceptive" to include the Pill as one. Now, a contraceptive prevents **implantation**, and not the heretofore literal translation meaning "against conception".

[4] i.e., energy is never lost; it all comes back to you.

[5] footnote from **Touch the Earth**.

[6] from a paper by student Lilyan Garcia McClure.

[7] She-Link has been reported to cause migraine headaches in several acquaintances of mine.

[8] Recall the myth of finding a baby underneath a cabbage leaf.

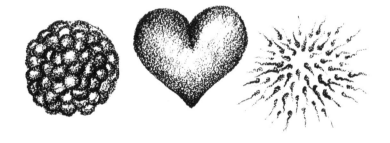

Gandhi & Margaret Sanger

The kind Anand T. Hingorani has granted me permission to reprint a conversation between Margaret Sanger, our American pioneer in birth control for the masses and Mahatma Gandhi, the Indian saint who proposed self-control as the best way to limit population. The dialogue appeared in the book Through Self-Control available through the Gandhi series, c/18-D, Munirka, New Delhi - 110057.

"Mrs. Sanger (hereafter referred to as MS): Sex love is a relationship which makes for oneness, for completeness between husband and wife and contributes to a finer understanding and a greater spiritual harmony.

Gandhiji (hereafter known as G): When both want to satisfy animal passion without having to suffer the consequences of their act, it is not love, it is lust. But if love is pure, it will transcend animal passion and will regulate itself. We have not had enough education of the passions. When a husband says, Let us not have children, but let us have relations, what is that but animal passion? If they do not want to have more children, they should simply refuse to unite. Love becomes lust the moment you make it a means for the satisfaction of animal needs. It is just the same with food. If food is taken only for pleasure, it is lust. You do not take chocolates for the sake of satisfying your hunger. You take them for pleasure and then ask the doctor for an antidote. Perhaps, you will tell the doctor that whiskey befogs your brain and he gives you an antidote. Would it not be better not to take chocolates or whiskey?

MS: No, I do not accept the analogy.

G: Of course, you will not accept the analogy because you think this sex expression without a desire for children is a need of the soul, a contention I do not endorse.

MS: Yes, sex expression is a spiritual need and I claim that the quality of this expression is more important than the result, for the quality of the relationship is there regardless of results. We all know that the great majority of children are born as an accident, without the parents having any desire for conception. Seldom are two people drawn together in the sex act by their desire to have children. Do you think it possible for two people who are in love, who are happy together, to regulate their sex act only once in two years, so that relationship would only take place when they wanted a child? Do you think it possible?

G: I had the honour of doing that very thing, and I am not the only one. I know from my own experience that as long as I looked upon my wife carnally, we had no real understanding. Our love did not reach a high plane. There was affection between us always, but we, or rather I, became restrained. There was never want of restraint on the part of my wife. Very often she would show restraint, but I rarely. All the time I wanted carnal pleasure, I could not serve her. The moment I bade good-by to a life of carnal pleasure, our whole relationship became spiritual; lust died and love reigned instead.

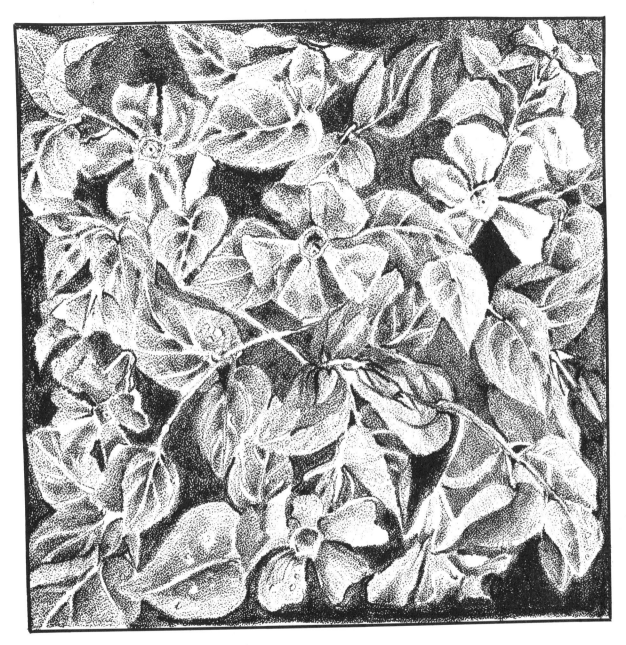

"Just what are the claims of Aphrodite upon our 20th century women souls?"
~Gordon Tappan

4

Anaphrodisiacs

Anaphrodisiacs are substances that dampen sexual desire - they are used when one's preoccupation with "getting it" or "getting some" become all consuming or obsessional. For many of us conscious of being on a spiritual path (and all of us are on one, whether we realize it or not), preoccupation with sex, or lust as it's sometimes called, gets in the way of our progress. Actually, there's really no where to go, as we all know, but be here now. However, within the illusion that there is a better world of spiritual consciousness, limiting one's experiences of sexuality has it's place. I refer the reader to Baba Hari Dass's writings on the subject, for his presentation of the traditional role of **brahmacharya**, as can be adapted to us westerners. Like Ram Das has said, if you're calling yourself celibate and yet walking around with a perpetual hard-on, you're missing the point.

There are other reasons why one might wish to be less horny. Perhaps your mate or lover is away for a length of time and you want to be "faithful". Perhaps you need to recover from some healing crisis and need to rest. Perhaps you are practicing natural birth control and want not to have intercourse during your fertile phases. And maybe you need time to be alone to feel your self apart from an intimate relationship for awhile. Along with herbs that traditionally dampen sexual desire, there are certain foods that should be avoided because they stimulate - garlic, onions, salt, and some spices - or because they're ennervating - such as meat, eggs (especially fertile ones - these when given to young babies and children can, in excess, force an early puberty). And along with foods, there's the media to be avoided - with its definition of intimacy between humans just about delegated to contacts below the waist. But this too, alas, is another story - as Babaji points out, sexual intercouse has no importance within a relationship when there's **total** communication.

The following are herbs used by various peoples for the transmutation of excessive sexual desire - and only you know what is "excessive" - if you feel tired rather than energized by your sexual encounters, this may be a hint . . .

I, too, beneath your moon, almighty Sex,
go forth at nightfall
crying like a cat.

Edna St. Vincent Millay

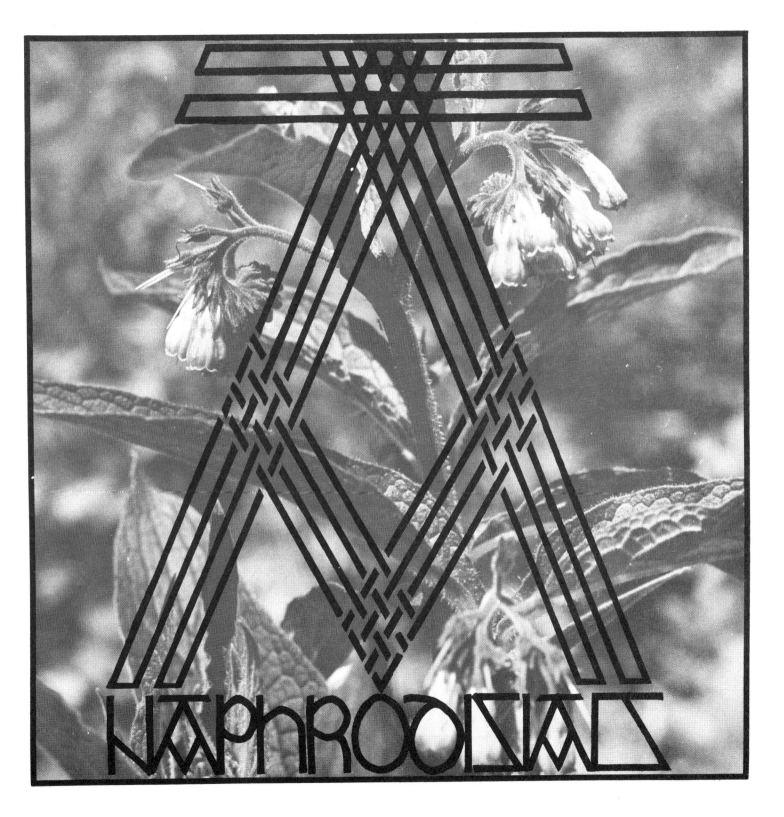

Anaphrodisiacs

Black Willow   *See White Willow.*

Blue Skullcap   *See "Infertility".*

Camphor   *Camphorosma or Cinnamomun camphora. Ancient herbalists ascribed great emmenogogic properties to camphor. Hermann. However, homeopathic remedies are negated by it - even in vapor, by exposure. Also used for hysterical complaints, and for "irritating conditions of the sexual apparatus". J. Rose. Arabians used it to lessen sexual desire. Use with care, if at all.*

Comfrey   *Symphytum officinalis. "Used by young girls to repair the irretrievable damage of love (ad sophisticated women virgin states)". Hermann. Known as "knitbone". As a douche, it cleanses the vagina and cures the whites. A leaf compress can be used for sore, swollen breasts. Comfrey contains allanton which aids healing of torn tissues. A sitz comfrey bath worked wonders after birthing my twins - in a couple days I wasn't sore even during intercourse. Put some in shoes and luggage for a safe journey. It's excellent for female troubles, and eaten occassionally raw in salads or blended as a "green drink" it's a fine preventative. We always grow a hedge of comfrey lining the visitors driveway - all our childbirth and health students are invited to take some fresh comfrey home with them. Called "Suelda" or Zuelda. Chicana midwives apply this mending herb as a poultice for vaginal tears.*

Hops   *Humulus lupulus. Urticaceae. The fruit have a resinous dust called "lupulin" which gives this herb its medicinal properties. It increases breast milk (which is why nursing women were advised to drink beer - nowadays, most beer is made by chemical process and non-nutritive). It's a cure for uncontrolled sexual desire and a quarrelsome nature. If possible, eat raw - otherwise, a standard brew. In pillows, it'll induce sleep and calm one, preventing nightmares. Babies and children appreciate this "nighty-night pillow".*

Lavendar   *Lavendual spica and Lavendual vera. Labiatae. It has been said that sprinkled upon one's head, helps keeping chaste. My friend Nan the midwife, always wears it to a birthing. "It helps the energy", she says.*

*Gather the potent flowers when newly open, but the whole plant is medicinal and a nervine. For treating hysteria, and in herb pillows the perfume was used to scent a room by the Romans to prepare for childbirth. Also to promote menses and deliver the placenta. A decoction of the flowerbuds can be used as a douche for leukorrhea. Lavender flowers, or **Alucema** aids a newborn rid his body of mucous. The Medica would trace a cross with the dried, crushed leaves over hot coals, to fill the room with this scent during birthing. For* menopause, a poultice of chamomile and lavender applied to the hurting part, brings relief. The oil is my favorite for hair rinses - I always wash (when possible) before attending birthings. Helps to prepare me for the birthing process. Sewn into the lining of a coat or jacket, it's said to prevent the Evil Eye from hurting the wearer, particularly children.

Lily Root *See White Water-Lily.*

Pussywillow *See White Willow.*

Rocky Mountain Grape Root *Kloss recommends this herb for all female troubles in many of his recipes - refer to **Back to Eden** for further information. Cited to decrease excessive sexual desire.*

Skullcap (or Scullcap) *See "Infertility".*

White Oak Bark *Querrous alba. "Tanner's bark". Used for women's troubles of the womb, leukorrhea, prevents nocturnal emissions due to excessive sexual desire and weakened condition. Checks excessive menstrual flow - excellent for varicose veins. For douches, steep a heaping T. in a quart of boiling water 30 mins. Strain - use as hot as possible.*

White Water Lily *Nymphae or Castalia odorata. "White pond lily". Used in the Middle Ages for the fluxes of the blood and for venereal problems. Also a vaginal douche for leukkorrhea–very astringent. Excellent for infant bowel troubles. Nymphaea alba. The name is "water-nymph" as the lily is pale and inhabits the water like them. The leaves are used externally for inflammations of the genital organs and rashes. The root for excessive sexual desire, "erotic burnings and insomnia".*

White Willow & Black Willow *Salix alba and Salix nigra. "Witch and Pussywillow". The Indians use the long slender trees as teepee poles. The Black Willow is used as an anaphrodisiac, to curtail excessive sexual desire. The bark of White Willow is used to treat menstrual irregularity, also.*

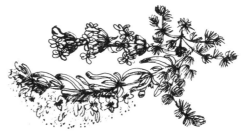

5

Aphrodisiacs

here the relationship between mind and body comes into focus. So much of our sexuality is mitigated by culture, images, fantasies, language and other "mind" stuff. The herbs chosen in this section reflect the need to treat the head as well as pelvis - and here I may as well add the **heart**. For in matters of sex, if the heart is involved we have the meeting place midway between the head and the genitals. The heart area is also the location of **thymos**, or area of the soul. So even soul is involved with sexuality - psyche and eros in perpetual intercourse. The result of this union is **ecstasy** and what better proving of the power of herbs than this pleasureable human experience?

As with **infertility**, the lack of interest in sex is best remedied by doing something about the situation. Herbs are the focus of our doings here in this book yet I do not mean to imply that other vehicles for inspiring passion are inferior. There are many ways: witchcraft, prayer, diet, (and attention to other aspects of basic health consciousness) body work, massage, psychology, and all its tools such as creative dreaming, journal keeping, plus poetry and music - but the best way I know of to excite the passions is to fall in love. Meditate on the planet/ symbol **Venus** and put your order in for a lover - when you give up seeking, it'll happen. This is offered not as a cut and dried formula, but as my confession*.

In the case of impotence, a re-mineralization is often indicated. We eat foods grown on depleted soils, and as one young man I know stated, he thought it was the funniest thing in the world to eat a **plant** when he was a teenager. Plants, **herbs**, will provide the minerals and hormone precursors so necessary for proper sexual functions. Clay has been used for this purpose - drinking a teaspoon in ½ cup of water every morning. Then alternate with a cup of fenugreek seed juice (made as a decoction): 1 T. per glass of water.

Sprouted wheat, again with the storehouse of Vitamin E - and also **vitamins** as found fresh in raw foods bring life and lively interest in sexual affairs. Dried fruits in moderation are also helpful, especially figs and dates. One Chinese herb, Elimecium macranthum, a species of barrenwort, is reported to increase a man's sexual potency.

* I'm indebted to Gordon Tappan, my Thesis advisor at California State College, Sonoma for this insight.

*But the subject here is women's impotence - often labeled "frigidity". Interesting how a man is 'not potent' and a woman is 'cold' when uninterested in sex. Personally, I don't consider this a problem, unless the particular person does herself (see chapter on Anaphrodisiacs). There are now many "pre-orgasmic" groups offered by experienced sex-counselors that may prove helpful in conjunction with using herbs. Primal therapy has also been found very helpful - if one is putting energy into repressing 'pain', then the other side, 'pleasure' is often put down too. It sometimes takes practice to fully enjoy sex - each woman has her own natural unfolding in regards to self as a sexual being. For some, it necessitates the birthing of a baby to appreciate more deeply the experience of sex. For others, it is becoming completely infertile before the barriers to enjoyment are let down. And for others still, it is the non-rational, eccentric and unpredictable meeting of a great lover. (Please don't infer the knight galloping unexpectedly on a white horse up to your doorstep - I don't mean this.) Every person can be a "great lover" - it's more a matter of the greatness of one's soul than appearance, technique, or experience. I've always valued sexuality and intuited that each lover I've had is connected with me, psychically, even after we've spent our passion together and physically drift apart. Consequently, Eros has valued me. For those of you attracted to the Eastern way of being in the world, you might refer to the **Tao of Sex** by Ishihara and Levy, or the **Kama Sutra** and the **Koka Shastra**. Ideally, sex is something that permeates all living things and experiences and is not an activity confined to genitals and bedrooms - it is an awareness of the unity of all. That is why sexual encounters are so ecstatic to my way of thinking - for a time we escape the illusion of separateness - of being skin-encapsulated egos. As ego dissolves, ecstacy comes in - or fear. Fear is very much linked with frigidity - the "chill" of fear: the contracting against the warmth of human contact. Look into your fears of sex - give a face, confront those ghosts of the past who gave you the information about being sexual. And, try some of these herbs and rituals:*

We'll want to wake up some dull senses most likely - saffron added to food is good and tonifies the uterus. Yellow Rocket sprinkled on salads or raw dishes is recommended by Dextreit as well as one tablespoon per cup of boiling water of Cow-Parsnip as a decoction. Here are some more:

Read the following herbs with soft eyes & a sense of humor — these aids go a long way, too.

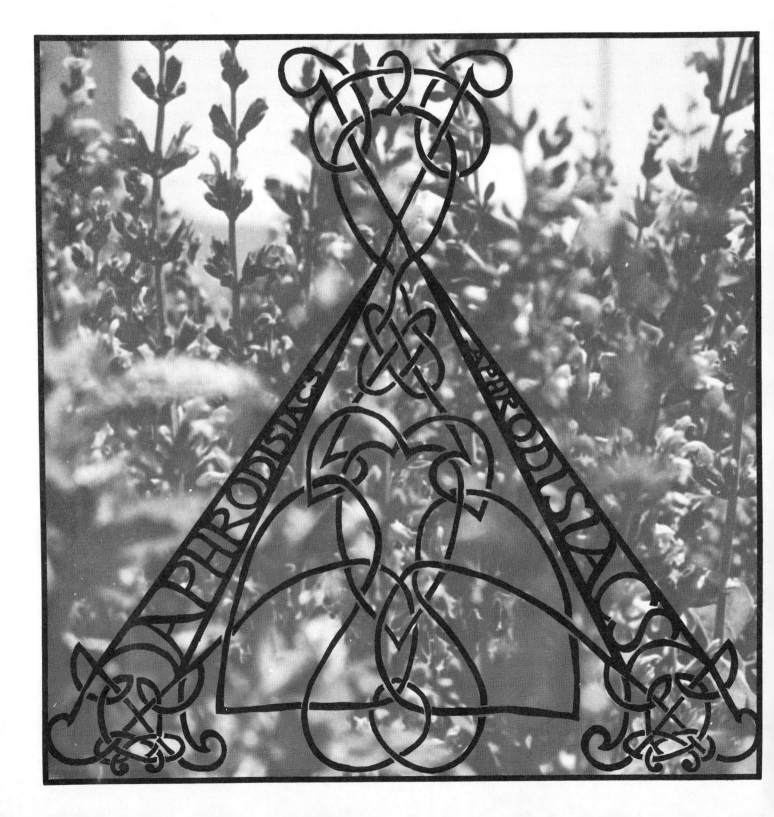

Aphrodisiacs

Cinnamon   *Cinnamomum zeylanicum*. "Oil of Cassia". Herman writes, "It stimulates the uterus, menstruation and uterine hemorrhages". Has been used for embalming in Egypt and in witch-craft. Was once more valuable than gold and used as an aphrodisiac in Medieval Europe. "Upon inhalation, the oil and incense is reported to act as a sexual stimulant to the female." J. Rose. The leaves were used to decorate the Ancient Roman Temples. "Taurus Cinnamonum". The Arabians valued the bark and used an oil to annoint the sacred vessels used in religious ceremony. Only the priests were allowed to gather cinnamon bark. Folkard reports that the ancients used the flowers in distilled water as a love potion. I use the bark to flavor our warm apple cider on winter nights.

Cotton Root   *See "Emmenagogues".*

Cubeb Berries   *Piper cubeba.* "Tailed Pepper". Used in medicinals and aphrodisiacs by Arab doctors. Kloss says it's an anti-syphilitic. Used to treat leukorrhea and gonorrhea and wind colic also. Increases flow of urine. May be inhaled or smoked for stimulating the mucus membranes. To drive away evil spirits, add cubeb berries to any incense. It's also an ancient love charm, used to melt the heart of the coldest one.when carried in your "conjure" bag. Riva reports the berries cause all you meet to look upon you with desire.

Damiana   *Turnera aphrodisiaca.* She is an old remedy for sexual impotence and has a rap for improving and strengthening the reproductive organs. Damiana is also a tonic for nerves. The taste is bitter with a fig like flavor. Take one tsp. of the dried leaves and pour a cup of boiling water over it. Dose is one tablespoon two times a day.

Echinacea   *Echinacea Augustifolia; brauneria palida; rudfeckia pallia; echinacea purpurea.* Also known as "purple coneflower", "black sampson", "red sunflower". We use the rhizomes in this one - the growth between the roots and leaves, and the roots. It has great antiseptic qualities. Cleanses the blood as well as destroying bacteria. Reported to stimulate sexual activity and have analgesic properties. Been used following childbirth to relieve post-portum diseases.

Garlic   *Allium satibum. Liliacaen.* "Ajo". Contains sulphur which produces oxygen and is antiseptic. A Muslim legend says that when Satan stepped out of the Garden of Eden after the fall of man, Garlic sprung up from the foot print he left. Baba Hari Das has said garlic is good for body, but bad for sadhana. It is a sexual excitant. Reported to destroy a magnet's power of attraction. Dioscorides, great Greek herbalist of the Roman army, called Garlic an holy herb because of its use for purification ceremonies in the temples. Homer says Hermes gave garlic to Odysseus to ward the beguiling spells of Circe. The gypsies worship this herb. Garlic tastes wonderful in placenta stews. (See "Placenta Recipes.) Use a vaginal suppository for infections, wrapped in a little cheese-cloth, remembering to leave a bit of wrapping to hang down in order to remove easily.

Mint

Mentha spicata. Used for treating infertility and lack of normal sexual desire. Also for suppressed menstruation and nausea and vomiting in pregnancy. Leaves are narrow, rough and very fragrant with a peculiar mint flavor. Flower are spikes of pale mauve and also mint-scented. "A wild water mint grows along ditch sides and was once esteemed as a cure for frigidity in both sexes. The Arabs drink mint daily to insure virility." - Baircli Levy. It may decrease milk supply so should be avoided by nursing mothers. Also called "spearmint". Makes a nice douche also. Yerba buena or spearmint and "poles" (peppermint) are used for colicky babies. A small jar of mint will protect against the biting of serpents, sea-scorpions and mad dogs. - Riva.

Orchis

Orchis maculata. Or chidaceae. See "Infertility".

Red Clover

See "Infertility".

Saw Palmetto Berries

Serenoa serrulata or Serpens. Specific for ovarian dysfunction. "Pan palm" as it's sometimes called, is valuable in all diseases of the regenerative organs. Sometimes mixed with damiana as an aphrodisiac. It seems to build flesh on wasting away genitals.

Vanilla

Vanilla planifolia. A known aphrodisiac; if the times of volunteered celibacy during your fertile phases are unusually trying, try to avoid vanilla (as well as all the aphrodisiacs and other sexual stimulants). Vanilla is an orchid and the most valuable one of all for herbal/culinary uses.

Wild Carrot

Daucus carota. L. "Another name, as is "Garden Carrot", "Carrot fruit", "Bee's nest plant", and "Birds Nest Root". Kloss reports it increases the menstrual flow. Use root and seed. Also classified as a diuretic, stimulant and menstrual excitant, increasing the flow of blood and helps in painful menstruation. During James I of England's time, the ladies would adorn their head dresses with leaves of carrots. The ancient Greeks called it "Phileon" and noted a connection with affairs of love. Galen thought if one dreamed of carrot, it meant profit and strength and the root could excite the passions.

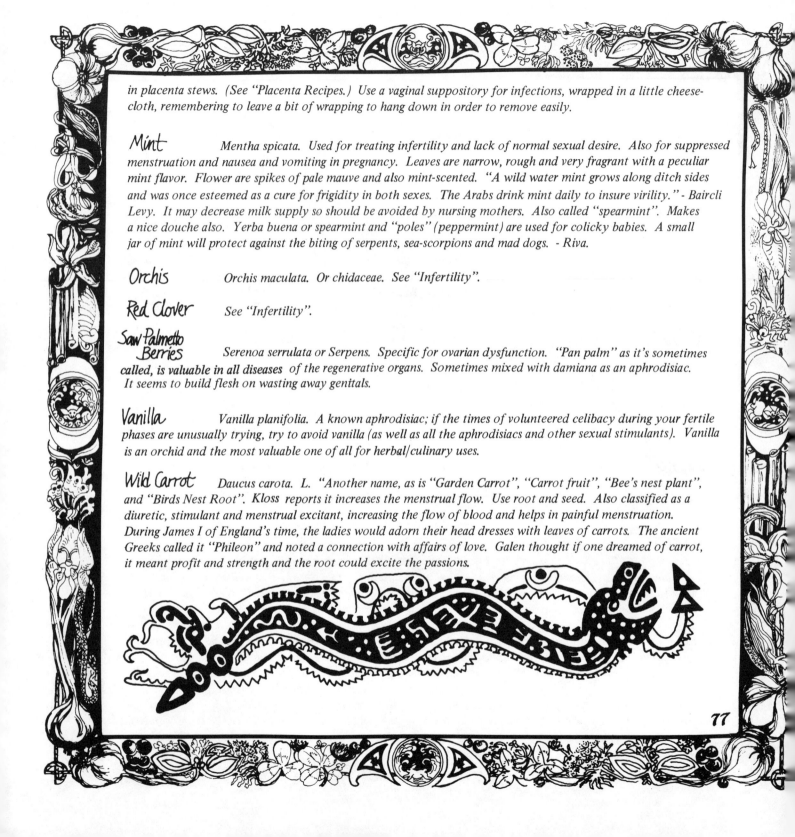

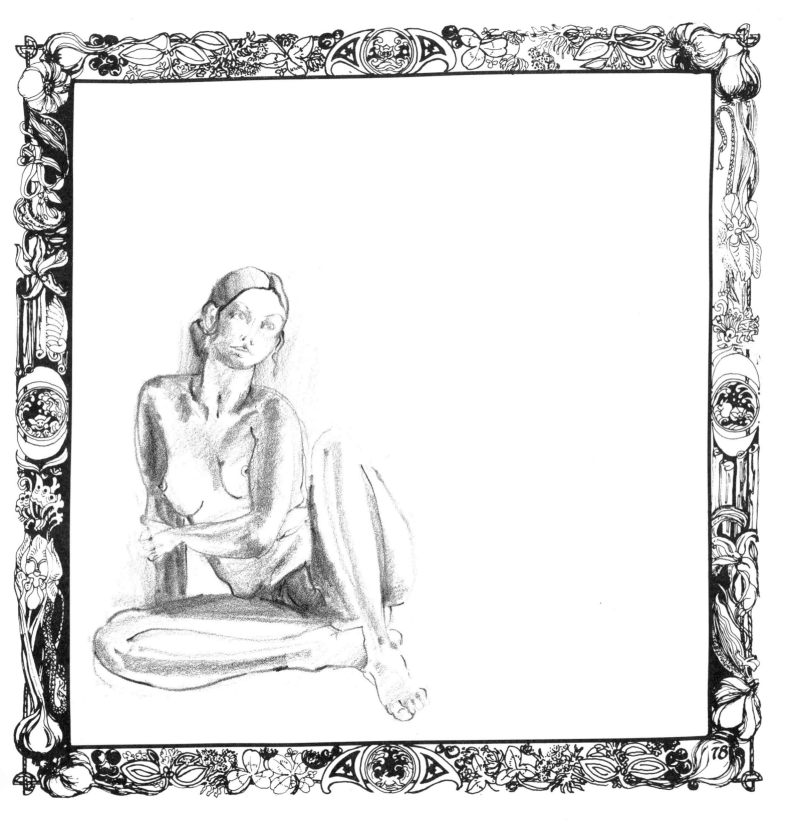

6

ḢERBS FOR the MINO

Marijuana

One herb, perhaps the widest spread and best loved plant of this decade, is Marijuana - Cannabis Sativa. It comes as a surprise to most women to learn that this plant is also implicated in birth control, women's cycles, and infertility. It was reported in the previous decade and before to increase sexual desires (perhaps, horrors, the actings-out of immoral lust). But more recently, researchers are finding other side-effects.

"Because of their chemical composition, marijuana and estrogen, the female sex hormone, may have a similar effect upon the body. Recently there have been reports of breast growth, lowered testosterone (male sex hormone) level and lowered sperm count in men who are heavy dope smokers. There have also been reports of **irregular menstrual cycles and infertility in women marijuana smokers**".[1] (Emphasis mine.)

Marijuana is used by many new-age identified women in ritual, respect and with love. It is an ally for some folks - a plant friend that guides us deeper into our SELVES [2] Always, in the back of my mind, Hari Dass's simple statement about grass reverberates reminding me that the permanent high is being with God, with the Goddess in my Heart.

"Studies on animals suggest that marijuana has a cumulative effect in long-term memory impairment in long-term smokers. I forget where I read it. . ."[3] Here is the first news I'd read to give us a hint, besides **Lunaception** by Louise Lacey, why many women have crazy, "irregular" cycles.

"There have been a few reports that some women who smoke marijuana heavily have **irregular menstrual cycles**, don't ovulate as often or **on schedule**, and consequently have difficulty in getting pregnant. Experiments on laboratory animals indicate that when animals take THC (the active ingredient in marijuana) they have difficulty in getting pregnant. Particularly if a woman smokes marijuana at certain times in her menstrual cycle - when progesterone, not estrogen, should be high - she might notice a delay in starting her period that month. Smoking good quality dope daily might raise the estrogen level in a woman's blood stream enough to mimic the effect of taking oral contraceptives. Caution, though: suppression of ovulation requires a daily input of estrogen, and if you miss taking a pill or smoking a joint, you could wind up looking like a pumpkin eater."[4]

As far as smoking Marijuana, or eating it goes, **when pregnant and after birthing**, let your brain - heart guide you. Listening to your desires mindfully now is very important. There have been reports of deleterious effects on embryos exposed to THC under laboratory conditions. In vivo, the usage of the herb in a body containing another body, may be a different story. I have observed the babies from marijuana addicted parents to have the white parts of the eyes a shade of cerrilian blue. Blue eyed babies are **very** blue eyed. Recall the **menage**, the psychedelic spice that people of Dune ate during pregnancy (and then would later birth blue-tinged schleras -

in their children, schleras being the traditionally white part of the eyeball). In any case, almost all pregnant women naturally lose an interest or taste for marijuana - to the benefit of their labor! Any smoking in the latter part of pregnancy cuts down on vital lung capacity and is infringing on the rights of the baby to a gentle and pranic birthing. And young babies need pure air - only use the smoke, any herbal and **pure** smoke, infrequently and for purposes of healing your babies only. Be mindful that a room full of adults smoking is getting any babies present very stoned indeed. Nursing mothers especially heed this reminder. We know from experience that flax makes for beautifully growing children - what do we know from our experiences about the herb marijuana? I'd love to hear your stories on this too!*

Ergot

Claviceps Purpurea "Demeter's Plant", "Siegle Ivre or Drunken Rye", "Tolkorn or Mad Grain"

A parasite fungus which grows on grasses and sometimes on cereals, especially rye. The spores, like mushroom "seeds", are invisible and have given rise to all sorts of mysterious theories about their origen. I like the fantasy of them coming from another planet. Upon inhabitation, ergot causes the grains to swell turning purplish in color or rusty. The color purple has been associated with Hades' hair and the robes of Demeter. She is the grain goddess and mother of Persephone, queen of the underworld. And just like any visit to the dark depths of the unconscious, sometimes her use is dangerous. She can give rise to a serious disease called "ergotism" if the infected grains are eaten. During the Middle Ages, one form of ergotism was spread through bread made with ergot-infected flour. The Christian community suffered St. Anthony's Fire, as the convulsions were named, in response to their attitude about the flesh, or body of Christ. And the karma for eradicating worship of the Gods and the Goddesses is still going on today; only the diseases have changed to protect the innocent.

In old German myths, it was told that when corn waved in the wind, the corn mother who was a demon, was passing through the field. It was believed that her children were the "rye wolves" or ergot.

Ergot may just have been the psychotropic drug used by participants in the Eleusian Mysteries. There's a wonderful book entitled, "The Road to Eleusis" by R.G. Wasson, Albert Hoffman, and Carl A.P. Ruck that documents this theory impeccably.[6]As recorded in the Homeric Hymn to Demeter[7], barley water (alphi) and mint (or glechon) were used as the sacred drink in the ceremonies. It is quite possible that the barley was infected with Claviceps Purpurea, as barley alone isn't noted for its psychotropic effects. And the mint most likely is pennyroyal, the herb personified as Hades' concubine in Hell. She was trampled by Demeter and made forever sterile for making jealous Persephone of her husband. Perhaps it was the ergot that evoked the spectacular sensorium experienced by the Eleusians, sworn to secrecy.

LSD   *In **Lunaception**, and reported again in **Moon, Moon**, the estrogenic effects of psychedelic agents such as LSD reportedly induce ovulation. We personally know a few sisters who did conceive during a trip (altered state of consciousness) though believing themselves infertile, way outside the expected time of ovulation. Since I believe that accidental pregnancies come from unacknowledged desires for a baby, it seems congruent with psycholytic theory that LSD can catalyze a pregnancy. So, even planning those orgiastic trips at infertile times of one's cycle may be a challenge to conceive **anyway**. I am still watching this one, carefully. LSD may be taken to see clearly one's world and it has been said that herbs for the mind, or psychoactive drugs have their place in the scheme of things. "Reality is for people who can't take drugs" - and I forgot where I heard that one also. However, personally I'd never take a psychoactive drug when pregnant, about to conceive, or still in the birthing space. Though, there are many pregnant botanists, midwives and herbalists who would, and do. Again, listen to your brain-heart, and the movements within, your **feelings**. If you feel comfortable making the decision to trip with your baby (baby getting a magnified dose due to her tinier body weight or mass), then make an **informed** decision. Refer to science, your own experience, and information coming from any channel. LSD is magnificent and for a fetus, it must be ultra-magnificent - but is it dangerous?*

I know that methergine, a derivative of the psychotrophic element in ergot, not only helps post-partum hemorrhage in newly-delivered mothers but produces "strange" feelings and perceptions. Methergine was discovered by Albert Hoffman in 1937 before LSD. The name for this ergo-novine substance is Lysergic Acid Butanolamide. It is the water soluble extracts of ergot which elicit powerful utertonic activity. While at work, the opus of consciousness, on the material which ergot provided, Hoffman discovered LSD. How interesting that the prima materia was womb contracting ergo - novine (ego-nervine) in order to expand phallic spirituality.

The use of ergot has been part of our gnosis for centuries. As early as 1582 a German doctor, Adam Lonitzer, was writing about midwives using ergot to precipitate labor. But Dr. David Hosack warned us not to use ergot til after birth and his advice was adopted to this day by most of the medical community. The alkaloids of ergot of rye are used as the base for many pharmeceuticals. Among the conditions these drugs help are geriatric disorders, circulatory and nervous disturbances, and migraines.

Morning Glory Seeds (Turbina corymbosa. Raf. and Ipomoea Violacea L.) have ergo-novine, the uterotonic and psychotrophic principle, as do the Mexican Mushrooms.

Peyote

*This is a sacred plant to native people of this land. I have never taken any due to a respect I have of proprietorship and ritual. However, I know of some women, not Indians, who wear a peyote button nestled high in their vaginas like a cervical cap. A peyote suppository, perhaps? Once I felt their presence, the alive and vibrating plant, in my astrology teacher's room. The peyote blended into the scene gracefully so it took awhile to locate the source of this heavy pulling I was feeling. When at last my eyes caught the peyote, the utter sensuality of this plant was overwhelming. I was floored. Just imagining wearing peyote in my vagina is almost too much! The women who **tell** me about this say that this is an exquisite way to "**suspend**" ordinary consciousness. And peyote have always looked like cervixes, which look somewhat like sea anemones anyway. The earth and the water - the succulent peyote.*

With all mind-altering herbs, the normal "set" of consciousness is broken for a time/space you are prepared for and invite. Taking these herbs can give parents an opportunity to feel their world as their children. An eye-opener, always. The first times I took LSD or Marijuana, my awareness of the world was akin to an infant's. Since then I have grown up from this primal space. Yet this quality of feeling fresh, one within the baby space, is still here in transcendent moments.

The ancient Greeks' tradition of women and their psychedelic plants is expressed in the image of Persephone. She is gathering flowers in a field with her lovely companion, Pharmaceia, which means "user of drugs". Persephone's flower is the "narkissos" from which we get our word for narcotic. The myth says that the underworld opened up and she was seized by the lord of hell, Hades. He abducted her to his kingdom to become his queen of souls. Mother Demeter mourned for her daughter's loss and that is why there is winter. When Persephone returns above ground, we have spring. And in the Mycenaean period of Greek culture, we have images of priestesses gathering herbs in fields decorated with vegetative motifs and crowned with halos of opium capsules. They would also hold a fennel stalk filled with ivy leaves, which have mild psychetrophic properties. The root "mycenae" is derived from "mykes", or Greek for Mushroom. Mushrooms are also thought to be engendered whenever lightening strikes the earth. They are a fascinating metaphor for the mysteries of re-birth; arising from the invisible, cold, and fermenting earth - the "mouldy other world".

Hecate is the Goddess of the Witches. It was her underworld experience that gave her the power over plants. She represents the dark connection with healing and female's trimurti with sexual energy. This Goddess suggests that we women healers regain our lost gnosis, our knowledge of the occult and use the tools of astrology, tarot, or other intuitive channels in our diagnoses and ministerings. For diseases have their hidden aspects, unconscious origins, and it is by honoring Hecate that we can come in touch with the subtler aspects of healing.

Teo Nanacatl

"Mushrooms of many species have been used for thousands of years as a healing, vision producing sacrament. Mushrooms are probably the earliest psycho-active plant to be discovered. Mushroom usage and worship has roots in centuries of native tradition. There are four cultural areas in the world where native peoples consume mushrooms for psychic effects: Siberia, India, New Guinea, and Mexico. In recent years mushrooms have become popular to people all over the world who are searching for psychic expansion and awareness. The Aztecs used Teo-Nanacatl in many ceremonies and celebrations to induce "The Spirits" to stimulate communication with "Los Antiguos" (the ancient ones) their ancestors and to help generate joy and laughter into special occasions. The Mazatec Indians of Mexico consider Teo-Nanacatl a sacrament and a great healer. The divine mushrooms are gathered on the new moon on the hillside before dawn by a virgin. They are often consecrated on the altar of the local Catholic Church. The all night Mazatec ceremony led usually by a woman Shaman (curandera) comprises long chants, percussive beats and prayers.

Often an effective curing rite takes place in which the shaman, through the "power" of the sacred mushrooms, communicates and intercedes with the Supreme Spirit. There is an apparent medicinal healing quality as well as vision producing effect in Teo-Nanacatl. Long term usage seems to induce longevity and increase stamina. Mazatec women are known to carry heavy loads weighing up to 200 pounds on their backs supported by a strap across their forehead. It is not uncommon to witness women over 50 years old carrying such loads many miles up steep hills without stopping, barefoot, in the rain on muddy rocky trails. Truly a phenomenal feat. In India, the ancient Vedic scriptures speak with great reverence about the sacred mushrooms; they are called "Somas." Vedic texts dating back thousands of years give many references to the Somas. Here are some translations of passages from the Vedas about the Somas: "Light has come to the plant a sun equal to gold," "Soma joins forces with the sun's rays," "This Soma is thy precise share, accompanied by the rays that are His in common with the sun," "Soma shines together with the sun," "Purify thyself with this stream by which thou Soma madest the sun to shine," "The Soma races against the rays of the sun, celestial vehicle beautiful to see."

Teo-Nanacatl can be safely and effectively consumed daily in the morning before eating or blended in a fruit or vegetable juice. Generally a daily dosage of not more than one half or even three tenths of one gram (accurately weighed), will induce a pleasant energy level, help balance the nervous system, and waken new intuitive dimensions, without disturbing one's ability to concentrate or labor at a profession. Daily non-addictive usage of Teo-Nanacatl can effectively assist in the curing of many illnesses and addictions such as: various drugs, smoking alcohol, caffein, obesity and more. The sacred mushrooms have a way of soothing nervous energy and enlightening the palate when used properly. On days of rest and fasting one will experience much joy in larger doses. Teo-Nanacatl is a blood purifier and has been used to summon the memory as well as stimulant to heavenly colorful inner and outer visual imagery. It is also very effective as an intuitive, creative and pleasantly stimulating guide for artists, musicians, dancers, meditators, philosophers, healers, monks, priests, rabbis, yogis, mothers, fathers, sisters, brothers, politicians, law enforcement officers, judges, presidents, doctors, lawyers, Indian chiefs, and anyone else *you can think of. Mushrooms reproduce by spores and spores are the only life form known to science that can live indefinitely in totally void interplanetary space without any elements for survival. After thousands of years of interplanetary existence they can land on earth and with the proper conditions and Supreme Will, expand into edible form and upon consumption, manifest Divine Experience, Light, Color, Bliss and Glory. How is this possible? Because Teo-Nanacatl is truly a form of the "Flesh of God." Godspeed!*

"May the long-time sun shine upon you. All love surround you. And the pure light within. Guide your way on."

The preceding was written on a beautifully illustrated package, "made in Heaven." The dried mushrooms are "soulfully guaranteed" and said to be 100% organically grown, nothing added but love. This package of love has an affixed value of $90 upon it, with enough sacred mushroom for 28 adults who weigh approximately 100 pounds, to experience an altered state of consciousness. Being obviously illegal in the United States, there is no manufacturer's or distributor's address on the label, and so I know not where to obtain more. I am not completely convinced that a daily usage of "Rainbow Light Healing Nectars" is serving Truth, and is so "healing." Yet I've never tried it as a daily affair either. What struck me in the blurb about Teo-Nanacatl, is the sentence about searching for <u>psychic expansion</u>, and the emphasis is totally mine. My intuition says that all this expansion, be it psychic or otherwise, isn't synonymous with goodness. Uncontrolled growth, expansion for the sake of satisfying a search, may be a quality of consciousness in need of a rest. Pathologizing this idea in the human body is called "cancer"-- the expansion uncontrollably of certain cells which bring about eventual contraction, and death. There seems to be a rhythm for "growth" or psychic expansion...My concern is the daily ingesting of psycho-active substances may be forcing it. And forcing the allegory, also. My understanding of "Soma" was that in one form it is a divine nectar produced in our heads that trickles down towards our mouths and eventually goes down the tubes into the gastric fire and is burned. That is why yogis practice jalandhar bandha, or throat lock, in an effort to collect a pool of Soma in order to taste its exquisite deliciousness. After some time of practicing regular pranyama, I was most fortunate to taste the soma, twice, and totally unexpectedly. It was worth the wait. My skeptic comes in whenever a daily dose is recommended and simultaneously called "non-addictive." If our psychic expansion must be triggered by sacred mushrooms daily, isn't this attachment? One can also be addicted to a yoga practice, I know--yet let's call a spade a spade. If the experiences of Teo-Nanacatl are so wonderful that we choose daily to eat more mushrooms, let us not advertise non-addiction. However, I like the story about the curandera, or woman-healer talking with the Supreme Spirit. What a colleague for one's practice! If all us women herbalists were to hold such consultations before administering, we needn't ever worry for mal-practice insurance, I'm sure.

Contra-indicated with mushroom use is yogurt, acidophilus, kefir, raw sauerkraut, etc., for the effect may be counter-acted. One cannot mix with alcohol, or any chemical drugs, for a serious negative reaction is possible. If one becomes extremely uncomfortable (usually due to over-eating), taking 1-4 grams of Niacin (a B vitamin)[5] will help, and more will bring about a normalizing of consciousness. More than 6 grams (6000 mg.) may cause the niacinamide rush-redness and hot flushing of the skin, usually beginning on the face and chest, maybe belly. It's harmless, but may be alarming if unprepared for the effects of massive doses of niacin. Also used to bring LSD trippers out and back to ordinary consciousness.

Why get high? Why expand psychic awareness? What's to "alter" about consciousness anyway? And just what is a soulful guarantee? I bring these questions to Teo-Nanacatl, and the goddesses visit me. From this experimentation with herbs for the mind, I realize nothing, have no questions answered, penetrate no further the mysteries. Attention focuses instead on the wound that doesn't mend and a healing does occur. It is for this "reason" that I include the psychedelic and psycho-active herbs.

Though LSD is not an herb, it is a widespread and well-known psycho-active agent. It is of our generation of test-tube babies and instant gratification, all well symbolized by the chemist's blotter paper; an invisible nectar.

"Everything that is essential is invisible to the eye."-The Little Prince. And so we finally come to what is essential, what matters. I first began searching for God with LSD as the introduction into the realm of the invisible and have come to celebrating with mushrooms the presence of all the Gods and Goddesses. Gods and Goddesses are my name for forces that move me, through me, and are not exclusive of monotheism at all. There are just many faces to the Supreme Spirit.

Teo-Nanacatl was yesterday's visitor, and having entered this abode of soul called Jeannine Parvati, is now written as first in my heart on the list of plant allies for healing. Again, please do not infer a prescription here. One woman's mushrooms may be another's......Your own friends will find you.

"May the Force be with you." Star Wars

FOOTNOTES

1. *Weiss, Kay "Marijuana As A Contraceptive" in **Co-Evolution Quarterly**, Box 428, Sausalito, CA. 94965*

2. *See **Book of the Mother**, Box 1441, Bakersfield, CA. 93301*

3. *Weiss IBID.*

4. *Weiss IBID. See page 216.*

5. *Sometimes, depending on the level of niacin in an individual, a reaction may be experienced with doses much less or more than 6,000 mg.*

6. *A Harvest Book, **"Ethno-mycological Studies No. 4"** 1978 Harcourt, Brace & Jovanovich. Highest recommendation!*

7. *Homeric Hymn, 2,206-11.*

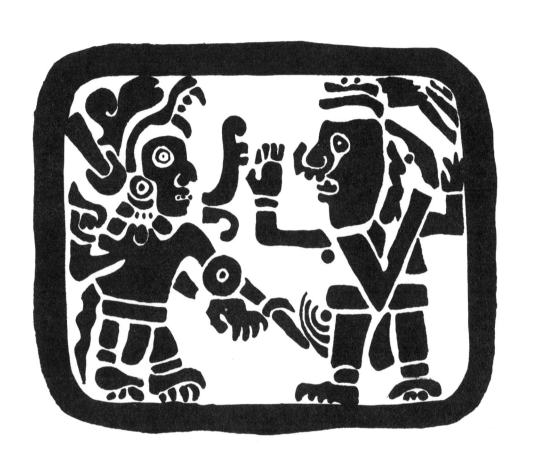

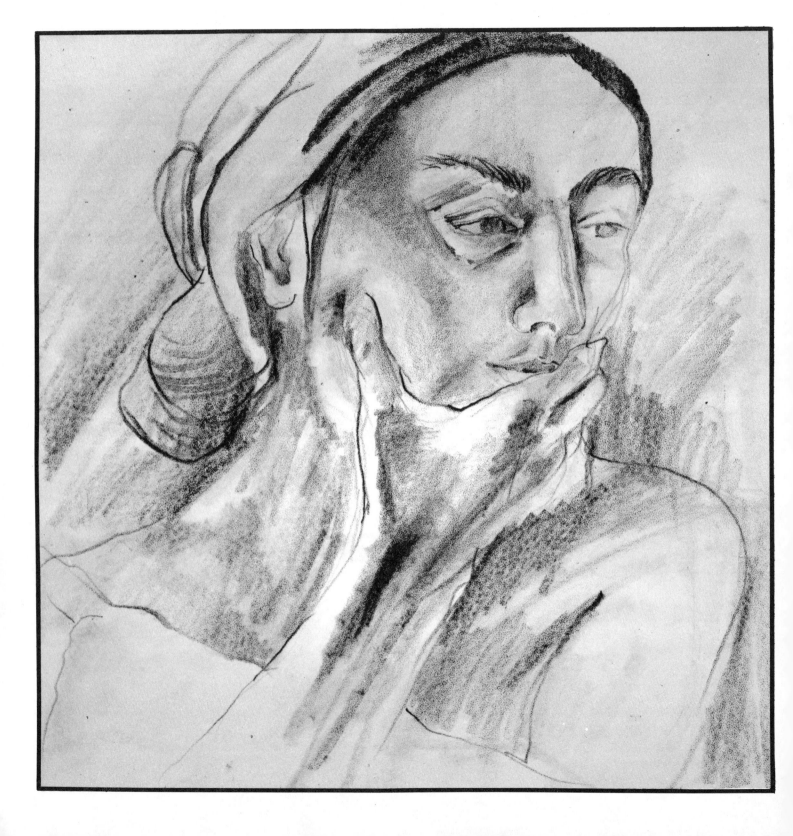

What's The Matter?

Basically it comes down to this **matter** of us as **women**, having less faith in the ability to heal ourselves. The word "feminine" is derived from the Latin "fe" meaning **faith**, and "mina" - meaning **less**. Somehow woman by definition has less faith; less than whom? Those church fathers who coined the word feminine to explain a host of female complaints and symptoms. The word as delivered by our patron here in the western world is "Thou shalt have no other images (Gods) before me - I am the One". However, how many of us here, upon realization that we invest as much energy, like religious devotion, to our pathologies, our illnesses and dis-eases as we would to any other token idols, find this God a wrathful one? And **does He punish** for our worships and sacrifices for the many symptoms our women bodies offer. The gynecologist offices have become churches wherein inititation, confession, sacrament and sometimes tantra takes place. In our initiation, we are asked to focus on our symptoms, give them a voice. The confession to priest-doctor is a ritual to which the doctor-healer can maintain his stance of projecting his "centered" good reality upon the confused and complaining patient/penitent. The sacrament can be a prescription, a piecemeal of advice and fatherly concern for our well-being - or it can be the sacrament of the Kali Yuga, one which is iatrogenic. Any weaving of souls, through the relationship of healer being healed, when carefully tended with love, and when the process involves genitals, can be Tantra in my mind, even if it's with a M.D. or whomever. Yet it seems harder to do tantra with a gynecologist in the process of healing because of this basic question of women having less faith in THEMSELVES and more in THE EXPERTS. *

What prevents us from being healers of ourselves and loved ones? And what is it about women that is still labelled as sickening? The nagging self doubts - our economy, patriarchial consciousness, Thanatos, Lillith, and let us not forget Typhoid Annie. We have a history full of words and images explaining away women-healers into those who are sick and those who cause sickness. For example, now we have feminine hygiene sprays, literally (translation mine), "less faith Hygieia spray". Not only do these sprays confuse sexual responses based on smell, but they actually cause reported irritations and infections of the mucosal membranes. Now who is victim here and who the one who causes deodorant and perfume on her cunt, perhaps the victim of socialization and other hidden persuaders of the patriarchy, but nevertheless doing any and all damage to herself. No one forced feminine hygiene sprays on us - consumers desire the product. We as women healers, have become the alternatives to Aphrodite, for our sisters who put beauty over health. In Hygieia they become one in the same. Coming back to our helplessness when our family becomes ill, or our selves - the Goddess Artemis (Diana of the Hunt and the Moon) may be a bridge from Aphrodite to Hygieia. And so we pay homage to the Grandmother, the Moon. O Hecate, it is you we become as we are set adrift when the moon is no longer in us . . . . .

*Who is a better expert about my own body than me?

.·····৶7ɛɛɛɛ·····

Self Health

Grouped within this chapter are herbs useful for treating all sorts of "female complaints". You'll find recipes for douches, concoctions for vaginitus, leukorrhea, uterine and ovarian disorders and all the herbs that are women's best friends. Not included, though, there are obvious overlappings, are the herbs useful for pregnancy, childbirth and breastfeeding. This section comes **first** - so that you can cure all maladies **before** the conception of your babies. For those of you coming off the Pill or other synthetic hormonal treatments, there's an extra seciton entitled "Balancers and Toners". There's useful information for any of us who would like a **regular** menstrual cycle and smooth menopause also.

I cannot emphasize it enough - good "gynecological" health is contingent upon general good health - and this is part and parcel of one's daily way of being in the world, down to thoughts and feelings, as well as nutrition and rest. Every women's book on health must include the importance of exercise, movement, and free flowing energy through the pelvis and whole being. Yoga for women is excellent for this as oftentimes, female complaints are due to poor posture - impinging upon digestion, circulation, body/fantasy, and elimination. The shoulder-stand will aid this, especially the half-form, as does squatting and dancing from a crouched pose. (Don't do the shoulder-stand when infected or menstruating - an infection could spread inward and upward and the blood will have a more difficult time flowing out, if you are upside down). However, this is a whole other book and in the meantime refer to **Prenatal Yoga & Natural Birth**, which shows and explains postures gentle enough for most all aspects of women's fertility. Now our focus is on health, the herbal way.

HERBS CAN HEAL. Therefore, their use is germane here especially for natural birth control practitioners. Using drugs, even in the form of synthetic hormonal therapies (i.e. estrogen replacers, etc.), WILL UPSET THE BALANCE of your body in ways science cannot always tell. In any case, the usage of drugs during healing crisises confuses messages our bodies are giving us. We are striving for clear communication in our relationships and within our bodies yet this can only be achieved in a clear psyche/mind. How can we know when we are fertile or not if we have recurrent yeast infections thusly obscuring the cervical mucous patterns? This section is perhaps the most important of our little book. By healing ourselves we are doing a politically and spiritually fine thing. Teaching our sisters how to take care of themselves may contribute to the cause of feminism, empiricism (or true science) and mythology all at once. We have been taught how to be "patients" and sick - we can un-learn our role as a "dependently ill" and "hysterical" person in the process of **application** (be it of herbs or otherwise). Each of us contains a healer in varying stages of awakening - call her out **now**, for the best political and spiritual *statement you could make, would be to heal yourself and someone else too. Let's begin with infections. I have learned a lot about sexuality from treating these over the years. My first experience of a bladder infection was during the pregnancy of my first born. Searing pain calling attention to my need to be mothered, taken care of, nursed. This was the last time I ever took antibiotics - these anti-life (literally) agents made me feel worse and my daughter was born with pitted and stained teeth, emerging months later.* Since then, I've investigated other ways for treating bladder infections. Advice is one tool - "Be sure to pee after you have intercourse in an effort to flush through any bacteria that may have been shoved up the ureter". Also, "Quit using those diaphragms! The bladder is irritated by vigorous sex with one of those cervical rubbers in place - and the pinch of orgasmic energy when wearing a diaphragm is on the same meridian as the bladder." The reader should refer to any other health writer for information about bladder infections - as both men and women have bladders, I've left this task to someone else. My interest is specifically on vaginal infections. My last one of these was also during a pregnancy - (How about this **quality of pregnancy** to make manifest all one's crises?).*

This time I heard the message and knew, I needn't do this one again.

*If you are prone to vaginal infections, a long, soft look at your life style, or way of being in the world, is in order. The most valuable approach to understanding one's illnesses is to give the afflicted part of your body a voice and listen to what you are indeed saying. Dialogue with your symptoms. An illness is dramatically calling attention to one's self. This is not by any means a new idea. The ancients too believed that diseases were messages from the Gods & Goddesses. Let it speak and listen to what your itchy and sore vagina is telling you. Are you aware of your sexual needs clearly? Horny? Or are you indulging in sexual intercourse, masturbation, etc., a bit too much? As women, we tend to punish ourselves for our sexual pleasures via our reproductive organs and it will take a major change in our political as well as personal cultures to allow ourselves sexual expression without painful repurcussions. Are you transgressing nature's laws, the basic ones - eating incorrectly (unconsciously) and/or too much? Not respecting your needs for rest, play/work, movement, solitude, and for **loving** relationships? Are you dancing enough? Vaginal infections are sometimes the result of a prolapsing colon - poor muscle and ligament tone from lack of exercise, and unnatural/processed food-stuffs, being the main contributors to this toxic condition. Again, highly recommended is yoga for women as many postures deal directly with restoring and maintaining intestinal strength and health. Massage is another valuable tool for releasing blocked energy in your body, specifically in your pelvic area when you remember to **breathe** - bringing your breath up to touch your hands during the massage. Let someone you love and trust place one hand on your belly, breathing deeply from her belly through her hands. She is grounded and protected, in any way possible that works for you and your helper. Her other hand is placed on your head and together you visualize the infection being burned completely out of your body, just smoke and ashes. **Wanting** to become healed is vital here. Sometimes we create an infection of the reproductive organs to get a rest from uncomfortable sexual demands we feel are being placed on us (by ourselves as well as other lovers). Seeing green light bathe the infected area, as well as consciously breathing healing energy through your vagina, feels wonderfully soothing. Pretend your cunt is a mouth, inhaling and exhaling, as you read now.*

** And, I was aware **not** to take types that would do this. "A mistake", the physician said.*

During a yeast infection, your body is in an acidic state and you'll need to alkalinize your blood. A broth of zuchinni, parsley and celery is good here. Supplementing with the vitamin B foods also, is for helping undergo the stress of an infection. Sometimes stress is what causes the infection, or allows it to manifest. This is how a daily yoga practice can prevent illness - yoga balances your being, down to the blood and the emotions, removing the causes of your stress (or at least giving you the strength to do something about the causes of imbalance in your life). A massage to the back of your leg just behind the ankle is helpful too. This area, a little above the level of the anklebone, contains nerve endings linking the female organs. Pressure here stimulates circulation while soothing and relaxing the ovaries and other female organs. This massage point can be used for other purposes than infection also.

If you are itching a lot, a pack of natural yogurt is sometimes soothing. Mildred Jackson recommends using "farmer's cheese" or cottage cheese, that is not wet, as an applied poultice. The **Handbook of Alternatives to Chemical Medicine** is very useful for other health information also. A word of caution with **dairy products**; douches, poultices and packs - some women are allergic to these. Especially the yogurt remedy for vaginitus. Make sure it's pure (no chemical additives) yogurt - goat's milk is preferred to cow's milk, mother's milk over goat's, and I hear that wolve's milk is the closest to human milk - make a culture out of some, if you can get it. After the birth of my first baby, I had so much breast milk that I seriously considered making some yogurt out of my extra.

If your itching is unbearable, make a paste out of slippery elm powder by adding a little water to the powdered herb. Apply it thickly and lovingly and then later, wash it out with a douche of motherwort tea, or golden seal, or oatstraw tea. Be careful when you douche - never let the douching bag be much higher than your pelvis, as this results in too forceful a pressure and could push the herbal water (which isn't dangerous in itself) up into your womb and or uretha/ureters. It's the infection that we don't want travelling deeper into our bodies, especially into our fallopian tubes. Douching, by the way, is virtually unnecessary when healthy and may actually upset the proper acidic balance of your vagina if done too often. Besides, douching washes away cervical mucus and you may be watching this as a message about your present fertility phase.

"If the condition is very obstinate, a warm water douche preceded by a hot Sitz bath will be found most helpful, and if the woman has a good reaction to cold water applications, a cold Sitz bath of one minute's duration may be taken first thing in the morning." - from **Women's Ailments** by Isa Anderson Kelso. pg. 47. For Trichomonas, strain a tea of chapperal and slippery elm, periwinkle and oatstraw, and then gently douche with it. You may also drink this tea (before you douche) and give some to your sexual partner to enjoy. Use prophylactics so as not to spread "trich" back and forth until you're sure both of you are healed. A garlic suppository can be inserted into your vagina and worn like any tampon. I have heard from women who've tried this to make sure that you don't nick the garlic because it stings **and** from other women to make sure that you nick the garlic so as to release some of it's healing properties. Wrap it up in cheesecloth lightly and remember to leave a tail like a string so you can change it daily. Garlic produces oxygen and sulphur and has been used for centuries to cure infections of many kinds. There is also an increased need for vitamin A and C as well as B vitamins when infected. These can be met through herbs and food.

Remember, only douche medicinally - meaning if something's out of balance already, otherwise, an alkaline diet helps maintain a healthy reproductive system. Diet also is implicated in the Ovulation Method or on any natural birth control method that relies on observation of cervical mucus. Those of us switching to a mucusless diet will find our cervical mucus changing dramatically too. Macrobiotic women sometimes stop menstruating, as do women who are brachmacharya and living in ashrams. Menstruation can be a time of renewal worth celebrating and enjoying as orgasmically as all the other aspects of our sexuality. But when you're in pain with a yeast infection, use Golden Seal Leaf, Comfrey, Sage (unless nursing as it dries up milk) 2 T. Acidolphilus, 2 T. apple cider vinegar and in one quart water place four T. of equal parts herb leaves. Steep for 15-20 min., strain and add the acidolphilus and vinegar. Douche remembering to use slight pressure so as not to push any organisms up into your urethral canal and bladder.

And from Culpepper's Complete Herbal we have the following: "Moonwort - the moon owns the herb. Moonwort is cold and drying more than adder's tongue, the leaves boiled in red wine, and drank, stay the immoderate flux of women's courses, and the whites." The whites being cervical mucus - one of the many messages our bodies give us about when we're fertile or not.

Motherwort tea helps decongest the body and is also good whenever the vaginal balance has been upset. Black cohosh helps to relieve lower back pains, as does walking barefoot on earth or doing the catstretch in yoga. And again most female discomforts can be avoided by fasting a bit before your period and during it on herbal teas and practicing the yoga for women found in my book[1] during your periods and during ovulation/lutein phase of your menstrual cycle. A women's yoga is in the oven now, cooking.

A few more words about the "Itch" or vaginitus, a catch-all name for symptoms of discomfort such as copious discharge that may sting or itch one's vagina. Women who take pills, birth control as well as antibiotics which upset the body's natural pH balance, and wear I.U.D.'s which make vaginal membranes more susceptible to infection, and/or who use spermicides (making one's cunt the battleground for the destruction of sperm) and who do not have "satisfying" sexual relations (whatever that may mean to each individual), i.e. those of us who are sometimes very unhappy and horny, are more likely to experience vaginitus eg. Trichomonas, yeast (monilla), or mixed vaginitis and bacterial infections.

"The Whites" - or Leukorrhea, is a message from our body about fertility. It is not necessarily a cause for remedial action via douching unless excessive (or actually the symptom of an infection - in which case you'll know the difference depending upon your degree of discomfort/pain). The whites are one way the body rids itself of excess mucus. I've included some herbal remedies for this condition if leukorrhea is a bother for you. An 18th century herbalist advises one with the whites to: "Live chastely; feed sparingly; use exercise constantly and sleep moderately, never lying on the back". If your discharge is excessive, it's a signal that your diet needs balancing. Check the bibliography for suggested nutritional reading. In our book on Conscious Conception, we'll be including a chapter on diet and fertility. Those of us eating macrobiotically or on a mucusless diet may find our cervical mucus drying up too! How do you practice the ovulation method of birth control under these circumstances? But this is the other side of the coin. Our focus now is on douching as a remedy for infections and excessive discharge.

Here's a suggestion for what is called a "retention douche" - women who have consciously toned their love musculature, i.e. developed their pubo-cocoygeal and vaginal levator muscles will find this easy. For beginners, here is the formula; the woman lays on her back, usually in a bathtub with the feet elevated on a rolled towel. Feel free to adapt to your situation. The syringe is inserted high into the vaginal vault until the fluid begins to run out gently. (See following pages for recipes for the "fluid"). The vaginal vault is filled completely with fluid, the bag is set down, and then the fluid is retained using the perineal muscles, as if you were holding urine in, for two to three minutes. The fluid may then gradually be released and allowed to flow out. Then the cunt is again filled, holding the bag up til the flow starts. Remember to be gentle and slow. This is repeated as before until the contents of the bag have been used. Retention douching takes longer, but it is more effective as the mixture is kept in contact with the vaginal membranes and the cervix longer, and acts as a poultice to draw on the uterus and vagina. For stubborn and severe cases of vaginitus, the douche by retention should be used two times daily. Once a day for moderate cases, and for mild infections, douching every two days is plenty.* Lastly, your focus on the itch with breath and mindfulness usually takes care of any problem if begun soon enough. Some well-deserving herbs are now presented as the cream of the crop for reproductive disorders. These are all best made into a tea, though douching could be considered. **Dandelion**, also can be eaten in salads and **Giant Solomon Seal Root** can be used as a poultice: **St. John's Wort**, one teaspoon powdered herb to cup of boiling water drunk three times daily - **Red Sage** with malt vinegar, one pint, to ½ pint of water and 1 ounce powdered **Red Sage**. Let stand overnight and take a little bit often during the day. Some herbs work better by flushing your organs, and permeating your blood fully. Manzanita is not only delicious in my estimation, but generally a gynecological herb. We're cautioned by Mildred Jackson not to drink **Manzanita** when pregnant though. Take one cup boiling water and add ½ teaspoon of the powdered **Manzanita** - steep for a few minutes, strain and enjoy twice daily. **Blue Flag** is reported in **The Handbook of Alternatives to Chemical Medicine** to clear up leukorrhea which is white and fluid. Use ten to twenty drops of the juice from bruised leaves in ½ cup of water, three times daily. Or one ounce of the powdered herb to a pint of water. I was glad to see my friend Dong **Qui** listed in the fine handbook. I like to take it once every few months for a short time when not pregnant or nursing. **Dong Qui is to women what Ginseng is to men.** I take very little ginseng, if at all anymore. It is better for men and I wouldn't recommend a pregnant or nursing mother of a female child to take any ginseng. Two more herbs are the very best - these two contain much natural wealth - hormones. **Licorice** has been reported to contain estrogen, and estrogenic like substances, while **sarasparilla** has progesterone and its precursors. I suspect they have many others as well as bits of male hormones too. I loved licorice when going into puberty - and sarasparilla in my teen years. Candy and root beer - make your own because to purchase it commercially is to buy into a farce; most use synthetics nowadays. The balancing of progesterone and estrogen is only ¡rudimentarily known. This is where my intuitions about herbs and listening to the effects an herb has on my body/psyche tells me more - like how much sarasparilla to drink, or licorice? Trust your own.

* See the appendix for more information of infections, douching and hypoglycemia or low blood sugar.

* Licorice should not be taken by women with cancer. Or women in the menopause who may have had cancer or are considering it as their style of dying.

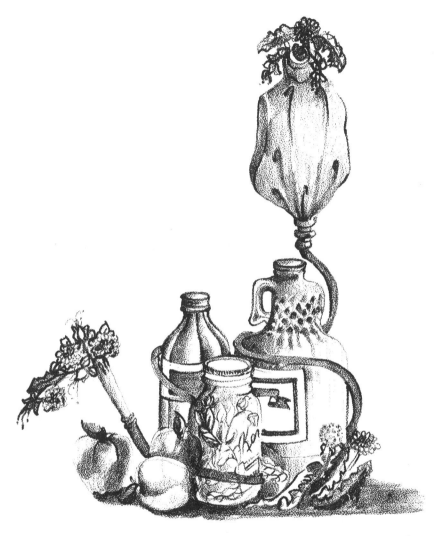

The last classification of herbs for birth control purposes is to retone, regularize and promote optimum hormonal balances. They are systemic, i.e., they will affect entire systems as opposed to specific organs. They are especially important for women experiencing major changes in their "regular" menstrual cycles like menopause, childbirth, the Pill, abortion, emotional and psychic upheavals, travel, radical dietary changes, celibacy or the initiation of a highly charged sexual relationship, and of course breastfeeding. The author invites you to mail us your favorite recipes (also see closing statement in this book).

If You're Coming Off "The Pill"...

Welcome back to your self! You'll most likely be amazed at how you feel now. No longer need you suffer the "emotional lability" so common with the Pill. An even temperment can be yours again with some attention to rebalancing and renourishing of your sexual organs and glands. Some medical people think that it might take up to two years to recover from the "Pill" but you can greatly aid this elimination through diet and herbs, and yogic purification practices.

Here is a partial list of the vital elements that taking the Pill interfered with: Folic Acid - so necessary for proper formation of an embryo, this vitamin is found in green leafy vegetables, fresh mushrooms, dried dates, and oranges. Eat fresh! Iron - sea vegetables, miso, figs, blackstrap molasses, and beets are some food sources. The B vitamins - these are the ones that will especially promote a sense of serenity: nutritional yeast (brewer's yeast) or live baking yeast on empty stomach, wheat sprouts, rice bran syrup, nuts, seeds and bee pollen. There are many more but this should get you started on correcting the delicate balance that has been upset by the "Pill".

*A healing meditation, concentrated on the area between your eyebrows and a few inches inside your skull is helpful, too. Also, all the yogic poses that revitalize the sexual organs - the centaur (see **Prenatal Yoga and Natural Birth**), the shoulderstand, the cobra, etc.*

We receive many questions on how one goes about using natural birth control when coming off the "Pill". It does seem that some women take a long time to establish a regular menstrual cycle with the accompanying mucus. The pattern to your cervical mucus secretions may be a bit eccentric until your system is rebalanced. In the meantime, know that the insertion of an I.U.D. (contraindicated if nursing - the contractions of the womb while breast-feeding can promote perforation and travel of the I.U.D. through the uterine wall) will also upset your hormonal balance. There are other forms of natural birth control besides mucus methods - the subject of our next book.

1. *Prenatal Yoga and Natural Birth.*

2   *The time I used the Pill (about 10 years ago) is looked upon now as a very unconscious period in my life. That is to say I experienced things happening to me, originating more from "out-there". Events came into my life rather than seeing my experiences issuing forth from within. I was guided by a visit with LSD to know myself and while at the peak of this consultation, it was time to take my daily Birth Control Pill. I held that little tablet in my hand, stoned as I never had been before, and just wouldn't do it. I couldn't swallow that ideology about fertility and female sexuality ever again. So I took a bite of the apple instead. Getting off the Pill is like the switch from buying waxed, reddened and poisoned apples in a supermarket to growing your own.*

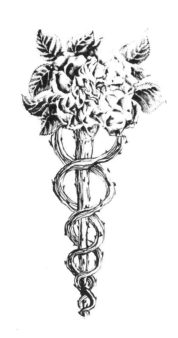

Balancers & Toners

The concept that a 28 day cycle is the "norm" and that pregnancy is an interruption of that norm is highly patriarchal. There's forever a woman changing inside of me. As soon as I'm classified, I will change again. I'm of the opinion that there is no such thing as an "interruption" - each happening is integral to my process as a woman. The cessation of periods by pregnancy, emotional/psychic experiences, malnutrition and/or spiritual purity, etc., are but more messages from my body about sexuality for me to understand. Watch out for "should" about "regular cycle" or now, a liberated ideal, the "should" aspects of Lunaception. Like, women "should" bleed on the new moon and ovulate on the full moon. It is the hardest thing to accept ourselves as we are right now - with bleedings coming seemingly regardless of any order or patterning in the cosmos. That is really O.K. too. The following formulas and lists of herbs are given as correctives - if you perceive an irregularity in your cycle as a problem, then by all means try some out.

Some recipes say things like, "Take five days before your period is due." Now just how do you know when that is unless you're regular in a menstrual cycle (meaning that for 6 months, you ovulated and bled predictably)? Most of these herbs help to tone the reproductive organs as well as balance the delicate hormonal systems. The Chinese say to take herbs for women's purposes late in the afternoon, with 3 - 5 p.m. being the best for uterine remedies. I like to imbibe female allies at dusk and into the night during the winter. Find your best time too, remembering to take them on an empty stomach with no distractions.

Here's a tea that is especially good if coming off the Pill or a pregnancy (either abortion, miscarriage, or nursing). It balances estrogen and re-tones sexual organs and glands: Take equal parts of: Sarsaparilla, Holy Thistle, Squaw Vine (mitchella repens), Black Haw, and Licorice. This is William LeSassier's recipe and I've given it to hundreds of women with positive results. Steep for forty minutes one tablespoon of the mixture to a cup and drink: First week: 4 - 5 cups. Second week: 2 - 3 cups. Third week: 1 - 3 cups. Fourth week: Taper off to one cup, then to ½ cup to sips. This may also increase your fertility.

We have to be free from dis-ease in order to practice any natural birth control method that works. If you have a recurring yeast infection that throws your cycle out of synch and obscures your mucus pattern, reliance upon the ovulation method alone is futile. Also, the use of antihistamines when ill dries up the cervical mucus as well - perhaps leading a person to assess infertility (dryness) when she might actually be quite fertile. Herbs for general health are outside the scope of this book - refer to the bibliography for our favorite herbals and/or seek out herbalists, naturopathic and homeopathic physicians in your area. After an illness, herbs help restore a balance in the female reproductive system - they also may help when traveling. There are some homeopathic remedies, usually plants, that have been diluted, shaken (succused), and thusly potentized into minute doses even for jet-lag. It's sometimes hard to feel confident of natural birth control when flying about the world - the zone changes

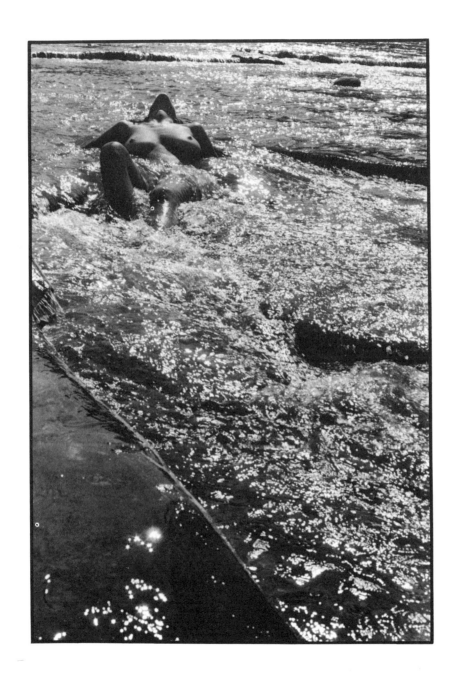

*are hard on our bodies/psyches. And if you go below the equator (or visa versa) then the cosmic or astrological fertility time must be re-calculated. More on this later in our **Conscious Conception** book.*

*To help aid regularization of your cycles: Five days before your period is due, take equal parts **Pennyroyal** and **Blue Cohosh**, two tablespoons per cup and steep at least thirty minutes. Drink in the late afternoon and evening for five consecutive days. Your bleeding could then begin at the end of the treatment. I have suggested this formula to hundreds of women with very good results. It is **not** abortive, to my knowledge, in the dosage recommended.*

False Solomon's Seal regulates menstrual disorders. Drink a root tea or infusion (it's listed as a toxic herb and therefore the correct dosage for your body/weight might be best left to an herbalist/healer to prescribe.) Smilacina stellata. (See appendix for an important letter about the danger of False Solomon's Seal.)

*White Willow Salex alba L. - use the bark to treat irregularities concerning the menstrual cycle: **Balm** Melissa officinales L. (especially good for delayed and painful menses). **Devil's Bit Scabious** Scabiosa succisa D. (also good for uterine disorders and vaginitus). **Mint** Mentha spicata and **Peppermint**; **Safflower** Cartamus tinctorius; **Senna** Cassis acutifolia L.; **Strawberry** Fragaria vesca; **Thyme** Thymus vugaris; **Wood Sorrel** Oxalis acetosella; **Rosemary** Rosmarinus officinalis L.; **Double Tansy**; **Rue** Ruta graveolens R.; **Cimifuga Root** (Black Cohosh) Cimifuga racemosa; **Valerian Root**, Valeriana officinalis; **Squaw Mint** (Pennyroyal) Mentha puelgium L. All these may be used as simple teas. The oils are much more potent - a cold-pressed safflower oil is good for salads but beware the oil of the squaw mint. Pennyroyal oil is to be used quite sparingly, externally only, unless you know what you are doing. Placed on my center- forehead, or third eye, the effects were intensely obvious within minutes. Strong uterine contractions were the result for about an hour. I am admittedly familiar with the nature of the plant pennyroyal, however and have always felt a kinship with her. In any case, pennyroyal oil is known to aid in the expulsion of uterine contents and for this reason is being used indiscriminately as an abortifacient by many pregnant women who find a technological abortion impossible. The irritation of the womb (not to mention the disquieting effect on the intricate hormonal systems) by an excessive use of pennyroyal, tansy or other abortifacients for prolonged periods can be in part soothed by using these herbs, says Laura Horton: **Holy Thistle, Raspberry Leaves, Blue Vervain, Nettle Leaves, Siberian Ginseng.** She recommends this to women who have used pennyroyal and or tansy **especially** use the formula sometime later in the month to normalize and tone-up the glandular system. Take equal parts of each and mix. One tablespoon of the mixture to one cup water. Simmer the roots and barks for twenty minutes; add leaves and blossoms, steep for ten minutes more. Again, the time for elimination for the female system, according to Chinese medicine, is 3 - 5 p.m.*

*More important than formulas, I believe, is the quality of relationship between your self, as healer, and the herb. I've mentioned that the best herbalists are also alchemists - well this is because there's **soul** involved in the process when you're an alchemist. Likewise, the best healers are witches too. "Womb is to birth like witch is to wimmin" says Z. Budapest. For too long we have deified **reason**, to the expense of **intuition - medicine**, to the fall of **witchcraft**. We all have felt the difference between a true healing in our lives and the mere cessation of a **symptom**. Rationalism,* who's greatest vehicle is western medicine (a' la A.M.A.), specializes whole, living beings* into categories of **symptoms** and treats people as pathologies. Witchcraft weaves whole, living beings into transcendence and cures people as participants. I'm for a blending of the two - the uses of perceptive diagnosis and empirical trusts. True healings benefit the soul as well as the body.

So, as you heal your selves and sisters with the following herbs, know that you are doing what millions of other wimmin have done since recorded time. Some of us were so powerful that we were literally consumed in the fire. Witches, wimmin healers (using mainly herbs as our ally), need not burn for the world's great sickness anymore. We did that in the Middle Ages. This is the time of Kali Yuga - an ushering terrible called the 'dawning of the new age'. Our styles must change to meet the challenge of the times. Let us be the gentle **women-healer**, the harmless ones. Let us know the great strength, and elegance, of healing with herbs.

* My gratitude to Harry Coulter, Ph.D. for this insight.

O Goddess
Ix Meklah Oyte
She who embraces
The dismayed one,
We dedicate
Our good work.

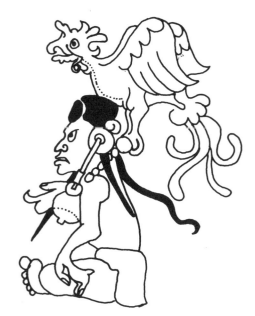

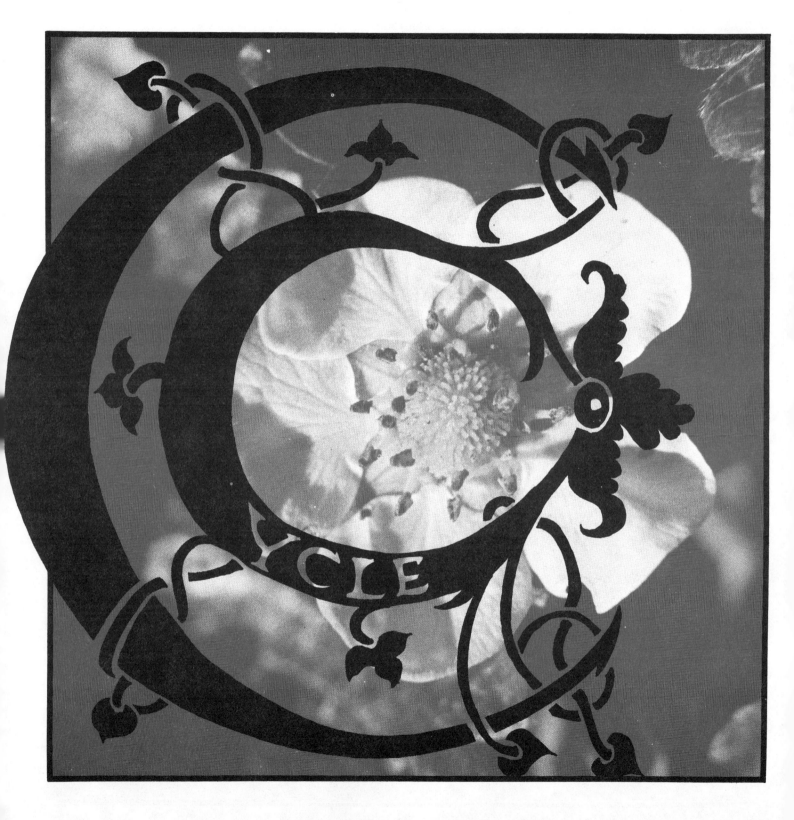

Herbs for the Cycle & Reproductive Organs

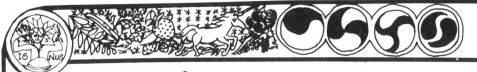

Acidolphilus

Though not an herb, a useful remedy for yeast infections of the vagina. Use a pure acidolphilus with apple cider vinegar, golden seal leaf, and sage. This makes a fine douching solution. We'll want to aid the friendly bacteria who live in our cunts to flourish again and douching, only when necessary with acidolphilus is a good way to feed our guests.

Alum

See Wild Geranium

Beet Powder

You can grow your own beets, dry them in the sun, and powder them. With a lot of binders and other nonsense, you'd have a fine "vitamin" and/or mineral tablet.

Bittersweet

Solanum dulcamara "nightshade". One of Circe's favorite herbs. It increases the menstrual flow, and is good for syphylis and gonorrhea. Place under a pillow, this herb aids in the forgetting of lost love.

Black Cohosh

Cimicifuga racemosa "macrotys". Used for pelvic disturbances, female complaints and all uterine troubles. Commonly known as "black snakeroot", she is used to bring on a menstrual flow that has been retarded by cold or exposure. Use the dried rhizome roots. Works on uterus to produce estrogene. Vogel. For the ovaries, also, and general womb trouble, says Kloss. Riva reports making a tea with a spoonful of this herb to a cup of water and sprinkling it about the room to prevent any evil spirit from entering. And for over 2,500 years, the Indians and Africans chewed the root to alleviate depression and calm nerves.

Blue Vervain

See Verbena.

Cimafuga Root

See Black Cohosh.

Colic Root

Gives tone and energy to the uterus.

Coral Root

Corallorhiza odontorhiza "dragon's claw", "chicken's toes". Very useful for treating scanty or painful menstruation. Will increase the flow. Dip in a cloth and apply to boils and tumors. Very useful for varicose veins.

Cotton Root

Gossypium herbaceum. Used to treat a painful birth by Alabaman Indians. When the root of this cultivated plant is air-dried, the properties are similar to ergot, but less reliable. Indians used it for abortive purposes. Again, let me caution the reader to not attempt an herbal abortion. Le Sassier has said that it is more traumatic on one's body than a medical abortion.

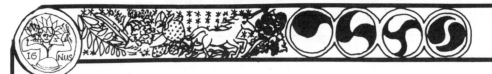

Cypripedium Root *From "The Female Regulator Tea No. 2". Stimulates the nervous system. Muhr. An ingredient in Formula No. 195 for spasmodic and painful menses.*

Dulse *Rhodymenia. "Neptune's girdle". Actually, a sea vegetable. She grows from rocks, ledges and other seaweeds. Very rich in minerals, very salty. You can rinse her first. I love to add dulse to soups in the winter for flavoring and added protein to our "garden cleaning" soups of land vegies. Raw, she is very strong tasting and chewy. My kids like it as a snack.*

False Unicorn Root *A uterine tonic. Included in menopause formula from Debby Ann and distributed at the Women's Centers in Sonoma County, California. No relation to the Chinese's Unicorn, She-Link. Also mentioned in Dr. Christopher's "Change-Ease" formula.*

Figwort *Monotropa uniflora. "Iceplant", "Indian Pipe", "Root Plant", "Bird's Nest", "Ova Ova", "Corpse Plant", "Convulsion Weed". Should be used in the place of opium and quinine. A teaspoonful of fig root and fennelseed, steeped in boiling water, 1 pint, for 20 mins. is excellent as a douche for inflammation of the vagina and uterus. Kloss.*

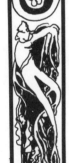

Gentian Root *Gentian lutea. "Bitterwort". Very excellent for female organs. Increases the menstrual flow and helpful in suppressed menses and scanty urine. It's the basis for gentian violet, a topical treatment for vaginal sores and infections. Since it's bitter, best combine her with an aromatic herb like mint. The root was named for an ancient king of Illyria, King Gentuis, a great herbalist. Valuable for many female problems. American Indians call her their "blue blossom" remedy. "Gentian Violet" is an antiseptic tincture and will stain. Take Tsp. of a brew three times daily before meals. Riva says a bit of Gentian placed in your pocketbook or wallet, protects you from pickpockets and purse-snatchers. Herpes is alleviated by application of gentian violet flowers.*

See Wild Geranium Root.

Ginseng *Panax quinquefolia L. "Panag", "Osha", "American Ginseng", "Garantogen", "Man Root", "The Fountain of Youth Root", "Flower of Life". Many miraculous claims have been made on this herb. Especially used in hot, moist climates as a preventative to many diseases. The root word panax is the same as the Latin, panacea. Very exciting to the gonads, endocrine glands, especially the ones involved with regeneration. Has been used as an aphrodisiac. Chinese herbalists have said to me that Dong Quai is better for women than Ginseng and to avoid Ginseng when pregnant. But afterbirth, Chicana midwives give it to prevent any infection. "Tartar Root" as it's sometimes called, was used by Indians to prevent female conception.*

Horehound *Marrubium vulgare. "Common Horehound". It has been used to treat menstrual irregularity. It will increase the menstrual flow. Culpepper wrote, "It is an herb of Mercury . . . It is given to women to bring down their courses, to expel the afterbirth . . . also to persons who have taken poisons." Superstition has it that*

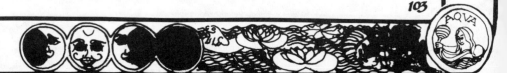

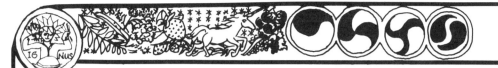

Horehound, placed in one's shoes, will keep away barking and biting dogs.

Laurel

Laurus nobilis. This herb is an instrument of divination. Aspiring poets may find placing a leaf over a blank page helpful. A packet of laurel given to a bride ensures a long and happy union. To make a wish come true, Riva suggests you write 700 times on 700 pieces of parchment, wishing 700 times on 700 Laurel leaves. You must start on Friday and finish on Friday night, then throw the 700 leaves and 700 pieces of paper into swiftly running water. To catch a thief, put Laurel leaves beneath your pillow and dream of the face of your robber. This herb decorates the statues of Asclepius. Make a mayfair crown of Laurel branches for all children. of spring. Decorate it with flowers and ribbons. Attention to the seasons and to our gifts of divination, seeing the divine in everything, are other ways to use herbs for health and happiness.

Marijuana

Cannabis Sativa. See "Herbs for the Mind".

Marshmallow

Althea officinales. Malvaceae. One of my favorite herbs for its soothing and relaxing effect. Can be used for burning and itching genitals, as a tea to drink, and as a decoction for a douche. Those marshmallow roasts by the campfire, once given up due to the list of ingredients on commercial packages, can now make a comeback. Indian Botanic Gardens sends a recipe for real marshmallows upon request in their Herbalist Almanac. Its name, "mortification root" comes from its ability to carry us through the campside ghost stories that used to scare us to death in the dark. This herb is medicinal from the roots up. Containing albumen, its sweet, mucilagenous flavor is familiar to us all. It is used for breast troubles too, as a poultice, and internally. It's good for venereal disease.

Motherwort

Leonurus cardiaca L. This plant is used with excellent results for suppressed menses. Taken warm, it increases the menstrual flow. A hot fomentation wrung out of the strong tea, will relieve the cramps and pain of dysmenorrhea. Jethro Kloss says it is taken with excellent results in pregnancy. A legend is to wear motherwort around the neck in a little bag to increase the flow of milk. My experience is that, with enough support and attention to diet, rest and love, the problem is usually one of overabundance of milk with my students. I've used motherwort for a number of years and have heard from many students about its efficiency as a douche for vaginitis when combined with other healing practices.

Mugwort

Artemisia vulgaris. The leaves are used in a bath for emennagogic purposes. It is a love-divining herb, and considered magical. The first time I put some mugwort in Michael's dream pillow, unknown to him, he awoke with a dream of taking LSD and meeting his guru, both very unlikely situations in his life at the time. This herb, taken with sage and yarrow, promotes the menstrual flow if taken daily. It should not be used if nursing, as it dries up the milk. Jethro Kloss prescribes, "It's splendid for female complaints when mixed with marigold flower, cramp bark, and black haw. Take a heaping teaspoon to a cup of boiling water. Steep 20 minutes, and drink 1 - 3 cups a day as needed". It was thought to be named after Artemis, also named Diana, the Moon Goddess. In 1675, Paul Barbette wrote that if a girl slept upon a pillow with mugwort underneath, her whole future would be revealed to her. A tea with honey is helpful for inducing clairvoyance and trances.

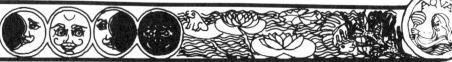

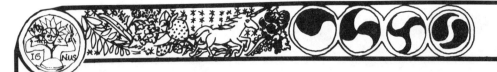

Myrrh

*Commiphora myrrha. This herb is written about on an Egyptian papyrus dated 2000 B.C. as well as in the Bible. It is good as a douche, with golden seal, for treating leukorrhea. It increases the circulation and number of white blood cells. It disinfects the genito-urinary mucous membranes. The ancients believed it to be the tears of Myrrah. There seems to be a connection between women's herbs and tears; our ability to cry is a gift, like the herbs given to us by the **Mother** to soothe our pains. The Jews used it in their sacred ointments with which the tabernacle was annointed. Also, as ordained by Jewish law, it was used for the purification of women. Myrrh was always burned in the temples of Iris, the Egyptian Goddess of Love.*

Parsley

Petroselinum crispum. Legend has it that a woman should always sow parsley. If sown by a man, he must be honest or thoroughly wicked. In Lincolnshire, there's a belief that if a woman feels compulsive about planting parsley, she is going to have a baby. The Greeks held it sacred, saying it had sprung from the blood of Archemorus, the Hero. It contains much vitamin A and C, iron, iodine, manganese and copper. It is also used for the treatment of gonnorhea and syphilus; says Kloss. "For female troubles, it's best to combine the leaves with equal parts of buchu, black haw, and cramp bark." Use the crushed leaves for swollen breasts or to dry up milk. I always have some growing around my front doorstep; all our children love to nibble at it, from crawling babes on up.

Pilewort

Amaranthus hypochondriacus. "Lovely Bleeding", "Red Cockscomb". This is excellent for excessive menstruation and leucorrhea. "Simmer a Tablespoon in a pint of water for ten minutes. Let it cool, strain, and drink freely", says Kloss.

Pleurisy Root

This is used for treating problems of the ovaries, to increase menstrual flow, and for burning, itching genitals.

Ragwort

Senecio aurus L. "Squaw Weed", "Female Regulator". This is one of the most certain and safe emmenagogics. It is good for increasing the menstrual flow, and good for leucorrhea when combined with lily. It has a very powerful effect on the female organs, and Kloss lists it with the best herbs for general female troubles. The root and plant have been used interchangeably. The Catawba Indians made a tea to hasten the birth of a baby and to check the pains of childbirth.

Red Cedar (eastern)

Juniperus virginiania. A decoction of boiled fruit and leaves was used to treat menstrual delay. The oil is a powerful abortifacient. Again, herbal abortions may be more traumatic physiologically than technological ones. Use of the oil has been fatal. A European relative, Juniperus sabina, also known as Savin or shrubby red cedar, is used to stimulate menstruation locally or systemically.

Rocky Mt. Grape Root

See "Herbs to Control Excessive Sexual Desire".

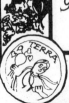

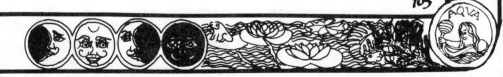

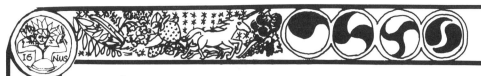

Sanicle

Sanicle mariandica. Umbelliferae. The plant's name is derived from a word meaning "to heal". It was a favorite of the Crusaders who recognized its power "to make whole and sound all inward hurts and outward wounds of man". De Levy. Also called "Black Snake Root", it will check women's courses if they be too free, and is used for gonorrhea and syphilis.

Senna

Cassis acutifolia. Leguminaceae. The leaves are bean-like. Remember to add a pinch of powdered ginger to each cup to forestall the griping pains, the sensation of hard adhesions breaking down in the bowels. Senna not only is a great laxative, but a wonderful aid for faulty menstruation as well. This is the imported Senna. The American Senna, Cassia marilandica, is not mentioned in connection with menstruation, but an internal cleansing would always help treatment of menstrual disorders. A legend reported by A. Riva says if one carries senna leaves, they'll bring forth the better qualities of those met. Also, make a tea of a spoonful of the leaves and cup of water. Set this aside for 7 days and then anoint the thighs of one's mate and he (or she) will be unable to "offer his sexual favors to others".

She-Link

"The Chinese Unicorn". Used with Chi Je Date, Ling-Shook root, and Gomsomcku leaf, it is advertised as a birth control pill you take only once every 6 months, by the Oriental Herbal Institute, P.O. Box 343, Vancouver, B.C., Canada. V6V-ZM7. If you change your mind, the antidote is 4 - 5 fresh or dried persimmons. The California would-be distributor stopped giving them to women though she personally had excellent results. Before she would give the dose, she would require a meditation on motives and clarity for the seriousness of the matter. Nevertheless, there were several pregnancies reported, so she gave the business up. She heard of no ill effects, though I have heard of side effects, e.g. migraine headaches. My personal decision is to let this "amazing herbal pill for longtime birth control" stay in China.

Solomon's Seal

Polygontum multiflorum. Excellent for all kinds of female problems. The rhizomes and the roots are used. It makes an astringent tea which "American Indians" used. (The tribe is not known to me - and I apologize for this ignorance, akin to calling whites "Europeans" without regard to their varying cultures). A.Riva writes, if you dream, and you want it to happen in your waking life, concentrate on the vision immediately upon arising with the root of Solomon's Seal between your palms. After this short meditation, put the root beneath your pillow and read psalm 32 before you begin the day's work. Leave the root until the dream has materialized.

Squawmint

Pennyroyal. Increases menstrual flow.

Squaw Root

See Blue Cohosh.

Stillingia

Stillingia sylvatica L. Regulates menstruation. The Cherokees mashed the roots, boiled them down, and the irregularly menstruating women bathed in the liquid with "devil's shoestring". (Tephrosia virginiaina L.)

Strawberry

Fragaria vesca. The leaves are a proven aid in preventing abortion and they also regulate faulty menstruation. The rash people sometimes develop when eating strawberries is a signal that excess acid in the system is being driven out through the skin faster than other channels of elimination. Information such as this has helped me to see the "allergy myth" in a healthy perspective. Being highly "allergic" as a child, I soon came to understand, via primal-type therapy, study of nutrition, LSD, yoga sadhana, and watching my own babies, that the allergy theory is one I need not live out anymore. The choice is always ours. Allergies "run" in families until we stop running from relationship.

Sumach Berries

Rhus glabrum. "Scarlet Sumách". Take equal parts sumach, berries and bark, white pine bark, and slippery elm. This tea is very cleansing and can be used for leucorrhea, gonorrhea, and syphilis. It is an emmenagogic as well.

Uva Ursi

Arctostaphylos. "Bearberry", "Upland Cranberry". Be careful! In large doses it is an oxytoxic. It is a disinfectant as a douche for the reproductive systems. It is good for excessive menstruation, gonorrhea, ulceration of the cervix, and other female troubles. Take a heaping tsp. in a pint of boiling water for 30 minutes. Then drink one half a cup every 4 hours. A good recipe for female troubles is to combine it with marshmallow, blue cohosh, lily root, and "queen of the meadow", *(Eupatorium purpurum).* Riva suggests when doing occult work, or as an aid towards astral projection, to place these leaves in an open bowl in the room. Occult means hidden, that which will be brought to the light.

Valerian

Valeriana officinalis. A German folksong reminds women to wear this "conquering herb" in their waistbands. Very good for nervous complaints. Mixed with pennyroyal, it will sedate a worried woman awaiting menstruation. It can also be mixed with blue cohosh; make a strong tea and drink three times daily for 3 days. It's a proven remedy for hysteria and used for women's problems. A favorite of cats, the scent, however, is usually unpleasant to people. It will increase the menstrual flow. Albertus Magnus, in his "De Mirabilibus Mundi" reports valerian to induce harmony between husband and wife.

Verbena

Verbena hastata. "Vervain", "Wild Hyssop". The sacred herb of the Druids, this was used in preparing their lustral water. Magicians and witches know this herb well. It's been used to prevent miscarriage; it is first boiled with shrimp for this purpose. Vervain is good in all female troubles; it will increase the flow of menses. *Verbena officinalis.* Verbenaceae, along with red clover, this herb was known as God's gift to man. In the plague years it was recommended as a safeguard. It increases nursing mother's milk, and was used in the Middle Ages to pledge mutual good faith. Vervain was used in many places to keep away evil spirits by steeping the plant in water, and then using the brew, called "Juno's Tears", for cleansing the house. What a nice way to make this necessity very special and important! The Persians believed that if they smeared their bodies with the juices of verbena, anything they might desire would be theirs, and any enemies would come to reconcile. Personally, I attempt to consciously limit my desires and confront my enemies with an open heart. It was a custom on Christmas Eve to build bonfires and dance, wearing garlands of vervain. Any young woman who gave her lover a garland was

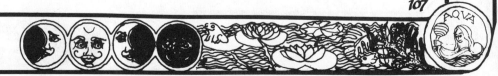

107

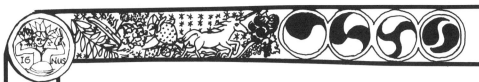

ensured of his fidelity for a year. And even in England, it's a belief today that a maiden who wears vervain and St. John's Wort about her person cannot be seduced by satan or evil. It's the Van Van oil of the deep south. There's 3000 years of tradition behind this magical and healing herb. Lemon Verbena is used to improve the complexion; make a tea with the leaves, take a clean cloth, dampen it with the tea and scrub the face full of pimples with it. Repeat each day. After nine days you should see improvement.

Wallflower

Cheiranthus cheiri. Galen says that the Greeks used this herb for abortion. It's used to treat amenorrhea, and in some pharmacopeias you will see the oil of keiri listed. It's by digestion of the flowers of this plant that the formula for the oil is obtained.

Walnut

Juglans regia. "Black Walnut". Herman recommends its use in treating leucorrhea, as a douche or injection. The walnut seeds (nuts) contain almost as much protein as a sirloin steak. A spirit distilled from the fresh walnuts calms hysteria and stops the vomiting of one who is pregnant. As an infusion, it is used to check mammary secretions. So, I'd suggest nursing mothers not to use it unless they want to stop breastfeeding. See Total Mothering, appendix.

White Horehound

See Hoarhound.

White Water Lily

Castalia odorata. Nymphaea. "White Pond Lily". In the middle ages it was used for fluxes of the blood and for venereal problems. Also it was used as a vaginal douche for leukorrhea. It is very astringent. It is excellent for infant bowel troubles. Nymphaea alba. The name is "water nymph", as the lily is pale and inhabits the water, like them. The leaves are used externally for inflammations of the genital organs and rashes. The root is used for excessive sexual desire, "erotic burnings and insomnia".

White Willow ~
~ Black Willow

Salix alba, Salix nigra. The Indians use the long slender trees as teepee poles. The black willow is used as an anaphrodisiac, to curb sexual desire. The bark of white willow is used to treat menstrual irregularity.

Wild Geranium

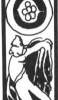

Sphaeralcea ambigua. "Storksbill". This was used with Desert Mallow by Shoshone women after birth to become infertile for one year. Total mothering (see appendix) no doubt had something to do with this being effective. Also known as "Alum Root", this is good for leukorrhea and excellent for treating profuse menstruation. In womb troubles it is used as a douche. A strong solution rubbed over the tits will dry up milk; rubbing just over the nipples will harden them.

Wild Oregon Grape Root

Berberis aguifolium. "California Barberry". Use the root for leukorrhea. As it's a good blood purifier, use it for chronic uterine disorders.

Witch Hazel

Hamamelis virginica. This is unsurpassed for stopping excessive menstruation. In gonorrhea, leukorrhea and the whites, use this as a douche. Internally, steep a heaping tsp. in one cup boiling water for

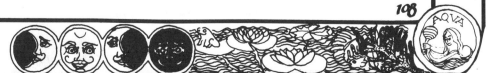

30 minutes. Take one or more cupsful during the day as needed, a large mouthful at a time, says Kloss. The shoots have been used for hundreds of years as divining rods for water.

Wintergreen

Gaultheria procumbens. "Partridge Berry", "Grouseberry", "Mountain Tea", "Deerberry". It's helpful in gonorrhea and the tea as a douche is excellent for leukorrhea (the whites). It is emmenagogic. The oil contains methyl salicylate, or natural aspirin.

Wood Sorrel

Oxalis acetosella Oxalidaceae. Used for menstrual irregularities and diseases of the sexual glands, this herb was the original Shamrock of Ireland before the Dutch Clover claimed title. The American Indians used it "to put the north wind into their hooves", by feeding it to their horses.

Wormwood

Artemisia absinthium. "Old Woman". Kloss says this is good for chronic leukorrhea. One species was used by American Indian tribes in their sweat lodges and baths to treat the menstrual disorders of girls. Use with great care until you know how it affects you. Absinthe, a powerful narcotic, is banned all over the world. It is made from wormwood, anise oil and alcohol.

Yarrow

Achillea millefolium L. "Milfoil", "Sneezewort". This was named after Achilles and brought to weddings to ensure at least 7 years of happiness to the couple. It's used for vaginal and menstrual troubles. It's especially good with mugwort and sage. If taken often, it promotes the menstrual flow. It is also used to check over profuse bleeding and womb problems. In the menopause, use yarrow as a decoction. In some countries, yarrow is used instead of hops to give sharpness to beer. The stalks are used when consulting the I Ching, the Chinese Book of Changes. I once was worried about the possibility of being pregnant. Michael and I had been practicing Karezza, or non-seminal intercourse, when passion got the best of us. We both experienced orgasmic ejeculation and I fell into blaming. "It's your fault", the loop that hangs up the free flow of being loving. So I meditated and consulted the I Ching. I read the changing line, "There's no fish in the tank. No blame." Sleeping with yarrow under a maiden's pillow would help bring her future husband to her in a dream. It's been used also to test fidelity in parts of England. The woman tickles the inside of her lover's nostril, and if it bleeds, he's faithful.

Yellow Dock

Rumex crispus. "Sour Dock". Use the root to treat syphilis., for glandular tumors, and as an internal and external remedy for "the itch". It's also called "garden patience".

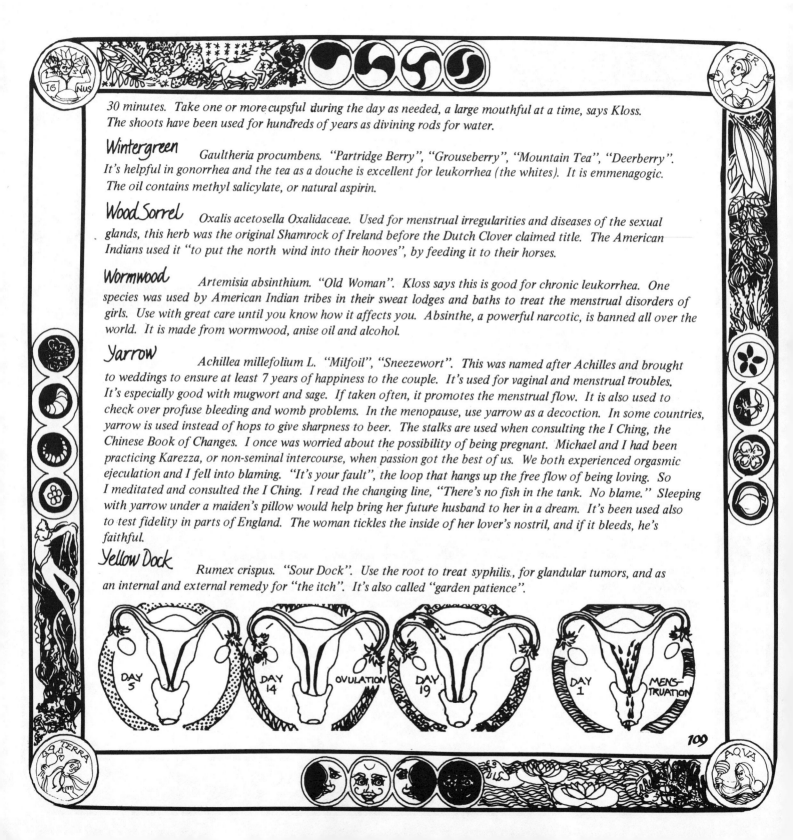

Check bibliography for books that have many more suggestions on how to heal yourself, and some will help you to even diagnose your own particular infection so as to choose the appropriate remedy. I'm aware that healing yourself, especially diagnosing one's own dis-ease, is an activity frowned upon by the American Gynecologists. But allow me to quote here a statement by their seat of learning, the American College of Obstetrics and Gynecology, distributed to their 18,000 bulletin recipients. "One of the main points is that the death rate from the Pill is lower than from pregnancy itself." This kind of deductive logic, absurd as it is, nevertheless is bought by the majority of so-called medical men-healers. Let us re-own our own ability to heal ourselves and one another. Herbs are but one tool in this venture.

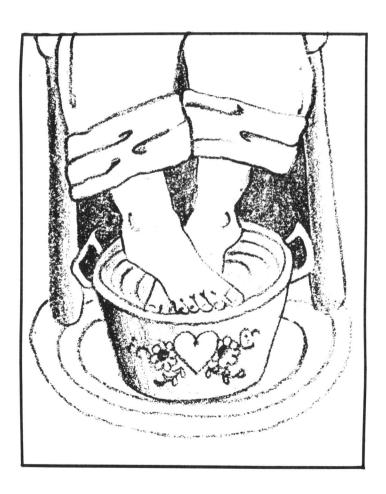

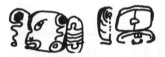

Dedicated
to Goddess
Lady Moon-
Birth —
IX·U·SIHNAL

Our Mother, Holy Mother
Grandmother, Mistress
Mistress of One, One Mistress

Moon Patroness of Birth,
Lady One Conjunction of Moon
She in the Middle of the Cenote,
Lady Sea

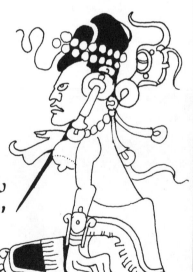

pregnancy, childbirth, lactation

As this booklet is but a chapter of a much larger book whose focus is on fertility and natural methods of contraception, most of our research went into herbal birth control and other gynecological considerations. To give obstetrical herbs its deserving place would result in a book much larger than we can afford. So I've included mention of all the traditional herbs for pregnancy, childbirth and breast-feeding that I know along with some experiences of using them over the years of caring for my family and being involved in the birth scene as a teacher and helper. We had set our principal focus on birth control initially and herbal ways to be healthy and to be responsible to that process of fertility; we had to share the best herbs for this most powerful of the meditative spaces, the baby space, also. Please read Juliette de Baircli-Levy's book, **Nature's Children**. And then don't stop there - trial and error, empirical investigation, experience - these, along with your children, will be your greatest teachers of herbology during the childbearing years.

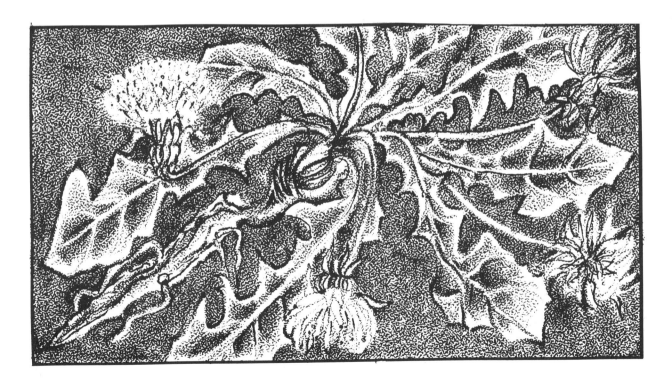

Pregnancy & GROWING it

This is the best of all possible times to begin your herb garden. As a tiny sprout of your love grows within, your days are filled with tender caretaking of herbal seedlings. The daily visit, under Dr. Sun's shining glow, to your herbal garden will help you develop qualities every mother needs - patience, tenderness, unconditional loving, plus discipline - just to get out there each and every day. This is akin to any spiritual practice which requires perseverance - good preparation for tending to the daily needs of a baby. Gardening literally gets you in touch with the Mother, our Earth. It is so much like our own fertile wombs. Enjoy your quiet moments among the herbal flowers - catching fairies out of the corners of your eyes - breathing the freshness of these plant friends. These moments may be your last of sustained silence for quite awhile after your baby is born - savor them. The coming of children are a bouquet of sound; yet silence has its own healing, a special healing.

It is the daily drinking of many of these herbs as simple teas which can make pregnancy and birthing one long unbroken meditation. These herbs feel much better than fruit juices or (heavens forbid) sodas, or chemical, sugared drink "beverages". Those beverages speed you up, are jangling and irritating to pregnancy plus contribute to the hyperactivity of babies and children as well. Herbal sun teas are especially inexpensive also.

Childbirth the harvest

In preparation of our homebirthing of the twins, I gathered as many kinds of herbs as might be needed - for any eventuality. I labeled each one carefully, according to use. The shelf above the stove, usually a poor place to store herbs due to the light and heat, had become a miniature pharmacy. Out from hiding in dark, dry places and into the birthing kitchen came the herbal allies. I also made some herbal ice cubes by making a brew, freezing it, and chipping them in case I wanted something medicinal to suck on during labor. It was August, and hot. I daily drank herbal blends that I'd made up - ones that felt good in my body. Ada Muir has a fine book on using those herbs that are favorable to your zodical influences. By checking out all the possible influences of a particular herb before I imbibe it, and pausing to understand which herb is right at a given time for me,

I am imbuing the healing with more soul-force. So, I like squawvine and raspberry the most. Try out your own blends - always realize that herbalism is a home science - watch, record, and share the healings. My weekly squawvine teas conjured up images of other natural women helping themselves to have the safest birthing possible. Do the best you can - and then relax to a delicious cup of herbal tea. Pregnancy is the time to get a vibration of LOVE with your baby. And to get to know one another, and just what it is that you are sharing. For one thing, now you have two hearts! (Or in my case, with twins, three!!!) Pausing for the cup of refreshing herbal tea will give us time to reflect on matters such as these - **and** *bring health to you and baby both.*

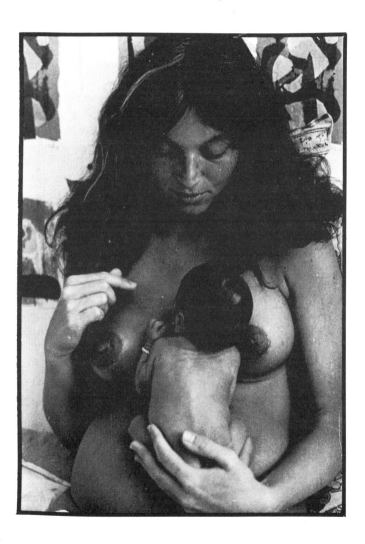

Placenta Recipes

The first time I ate placenta was after a very powerful birthing. The mother ate some raw first; and then let me take some into the kitchen for fixing. My experience of this slab of meat was amazing. I had never felt such life-force present in meat before. For one obvious reason, that this food came to us without killing. No animal suffered or was brought down by someone else, higher up in the hierarchial food chain. Not exactly dog eat dog ... The mother reported a painless childbirth and was not afraid. This meat still felt very much alive to me as I began to slice it and saute it in garlic and oil. I used the rosemary and basil growing outside the kitchen door, if memory serves me correctly. The serenity in the meat enveloped me as it cooked, and I recalled the birthing. The mother's meditation was unbroken for the entire process - another perfect birthing (as they all are). By the time the placenta was tender, the birthday party members were very hungry, and exhausted. After the supper, eaten in a glowing silence, everyone was energized, very much re-vitalized. So this is why mother animals eat their placentas, even my "vegetarian" goats, I thought. Adelle Davis's theoretical statement that the ideal food for humans, is other humans, finally made sense. Notwithstanding, the first time I ate placenta has also been my last time - though I've been around a number of stews. Guess I just lost my taste.

In Brazil, the Moon is believed to be the creator of vegetables, and is in fact called, "the mother of plants". What connects us, roots us to this mythology, is our placentas. The King of a Brazilian tribe of peoples (as reported in the **Golden Bough**) places his own placenta out in the open, immediately after the light of the new moon. It is said to be a way of re-vitalizing the King. Frazier (Mentor Books, 1964) writes that this ceremony, by means of the moon's waxing influences, acts upon the external soul of the King, symbolized by his placenta. An external soul. At some hospitals, the obstetrical nurses ask the newly delivered couple if they'd like a doggie bag for their placenta in case they'd like to take their's home with them. An external soul... Once I came to my mailbox, reached in, to find my hand grasping a bloody placenta in a soaked paper bag. One of my childbirth students, remembering that I'd wanted a placenta with which to instruct my student midwives, gifted me with hers - but not finding me at home, deposited it in the next likely place - my mailbox. I'm just glad I found it before my mailman.

We put our first placenta, Loi's, in a bottle of formulin, a chemical preservative. Being conscientious students of the body, the opportunity for our daughter to one day study her own placenta was appealing to us. It was later destroyed in a fire. I was relieved - it was a ghastly thing by then and our little girl was more interested in learning how to fly and have magic than study cadavers.

With our second placenta, Oceana & Cheyenne's one fused placenta, we experimented with the Lotus Birthing.

When I was pregnant with the twins, a woman appeared one day on my doorstep with this, as an opening,

"He! The Tribal Healing Council sent me to you. I am a psychic, a clairvoyant, and have envisioned your twins being of the Lotus Birthing." "Wow", I thought, "this is alot better than someone trying to sell me brushes." And I welcomed her in. She proceeded to tell me the precepts of this New-Age way of bringing souls into our world. All the time she spoke, my eyes were seeing her son, Trimurti, as the avatar. He is a beautiful child, no doubt about that, but back then I saw him with the eyes-of-full-pregnancy - the ones that see every mother as Madonna and every child the Christ. By the time she had explained that Trimurti was her proof of what the Lotus birthing can do for humanity, I'd promised to do likewise for my children, and all others I helped birth. Basically, it meant that our second placenta was placed in a pyramid. Well, that's one step up from a jar of poison/preserver, one might say. Perhaps it was even cosmic. In any case, in the Lotus Birth, the umbilical cord is allowed to dry up and drop off naturally, usually within days. No cutting - that is the first violence (aside from the "conventional" childbirth in hospitals as usually "practiced") committed against our babies. Circumcision is the second. (See appendix.) So in order to retain the connection of family harmony, we chose not to sever the umbilical cords of the babies and therefore carry around not only two babies, but their placenta as well!* Well, this being August, and very hot in Northern California, we had to put the quickly rotting placenta under a pyramid to delay the spoilage. But the placenta was much too big for the cover to fit tightly - and the inevitable decay set in. Michael and I each threw a line of the I CHING asking if cutting the umbilicus now would be an act of violence in our family. We read the hexagram "The Family - all the lines in the right place." And so fifteen hours after birth, we each cut the cords of our daughters. And I did feel the tiniest snip of Kundalini in my spine, at the moment of severance. Yogi midwives, here is something else for you to watch - is a psychic cord cut also with the umbilicus?

Well, our second placenta, unnamed, ultimately was buried in our garden, which isn't at all an original idea. Friends of ours had buried their two under trees that they planted and held sacred to their children. Sequoya and Willow were the trees and their son and daughter. I planted a friend's placenta in the center of a mandala vegetable/flower garden plot one full moon years ago.

*Namings, by the way, of our children are reflecting the return to more nature-centered life-styles. Many herb and flower names are becoming very popular as I watch the new-age babies come in. Lavender, Sage, Rose, Heather, Lily, Juniper, and even my friend Raspberry - as well as all other natural phenomenom - Sky, Tree, Forest, Luna, and I must confess to naming my second daughter after the Ocean, Violet, her middle name, and my third daughter's second name is Coral, again after the color of this sea. Instead of little "Johnny and Susie", it is "Rainbow and Cloud". In **Titters: The First Collection of Humor by Women**, there's a hilarious parody on this trend - it's entitled, "The Whole Birth Catalog".*

---

* We'd first seen this many years previous when friends of ours proudly showed off their new daughter "Ginger" and their placenta, "Sam".

Nursing and the Green Tit

What more perfect drink for the thirsty nursing mother than herbal teas? With my nursing of the twins for three years, I have tried most all ways to have an adequate fluid intake and energy supply. **Borage** is my all time favorite, hands down. It is beautifully easy to grow and that blue-purple color of its flowers gladdens even the driest heart. But we are told, if anything at all, to drink beer - for nourishment, and fluid, and to relax so that our milk can let-down the richer stuff. How nice that herbs provide an alternative that match all conditions. One of the mythological connections here is the herb **Hops**, used for brewing good tasting beer. However, most beer nowadays is processed by chemicals, so that the brewer's yeast (so valuable for abundant milk supply) is best obtained through the health food store. Natural B Vitamins aren't found in domestic beers and lots of the imported brews too.

Herbs can help to relax us as well as providing nutrition, the extra energy needed when nursing our babies. Only breastfeeding mothers can know the drought and uptightness we feel when extremely thirsty. Always have a little quenching tea ready for nursing friends too. And whenever you want to treat a baby medicinally, have the nursing mother drink the remedy - she'll pass along the benefits in her milk. You can also give a baby an herbal bath, allowing the essences to be drunk in by open pores. They have yet to close down to an inhospitable or unloving environment and can still drink in what they need through their skin. The more polluted your environment, the more in need you **both** are of saunas and herbal baths to re-open your pores, in skin contracted against the toxins, within and without. The process of nursing is a flowing one - all manners of things flow through the breastmilk - it is up to you to discriminate which substances build health and which do not. Nursing mothers cannot take drugs - they pass through the milk. Her body, when ill anyway, passes immunity to the illness through the milk, to her baby. That is why a breast-fed baby is often the only one in a family not to become sick when illness stops the rest of the members cold. A breastfeeding mother **can** take most herbal remedies however, feeling safe that her baby is only benefited by most herbs, in the dosages found in milk.

And then, the throes of weaning, when you know that **time** has come to end this way of loving, via the green tit; herbs may again befriend you. There are some which dry up the milk - others which help with sore and inflamed breasts. And still others to help you, the mama, let go **your** need to nourish in this way.

Once again, this is presented as a partial list of herbs for pregnancy, birth and lactation. All you really need are a few friends here - growing outside the doorstep - a few flowers by the kitchen sink. Good friends in the plant kingdom will serve you well your entire time as a householder - and knowing a couple in depth can enrich the health of you and baby immensely. Going back to my example of **Borage** - not only does it make primo milk (calcium and phosphorus is the right ratio for my nursing requirements), but she also helps when feeling depressed or sad to end a nursing relationship. In time, you will find yours - and then pass along the secrets to your daughters **and our herbal lore will grow and grow!**

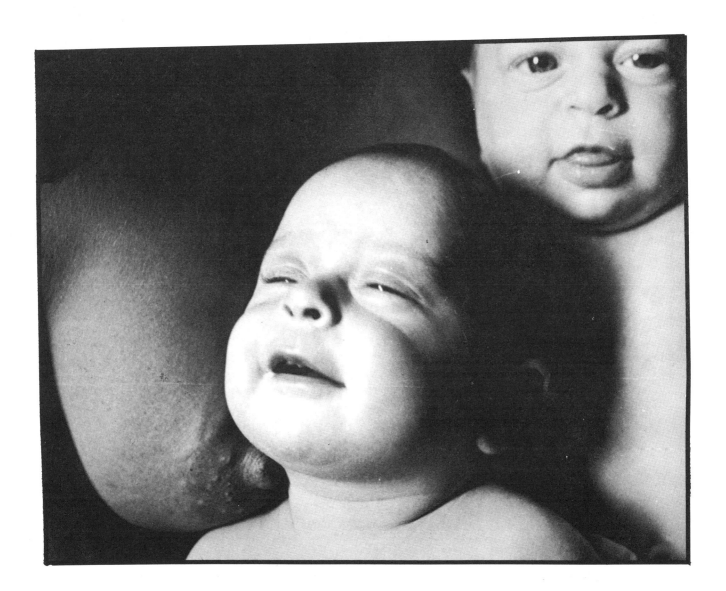

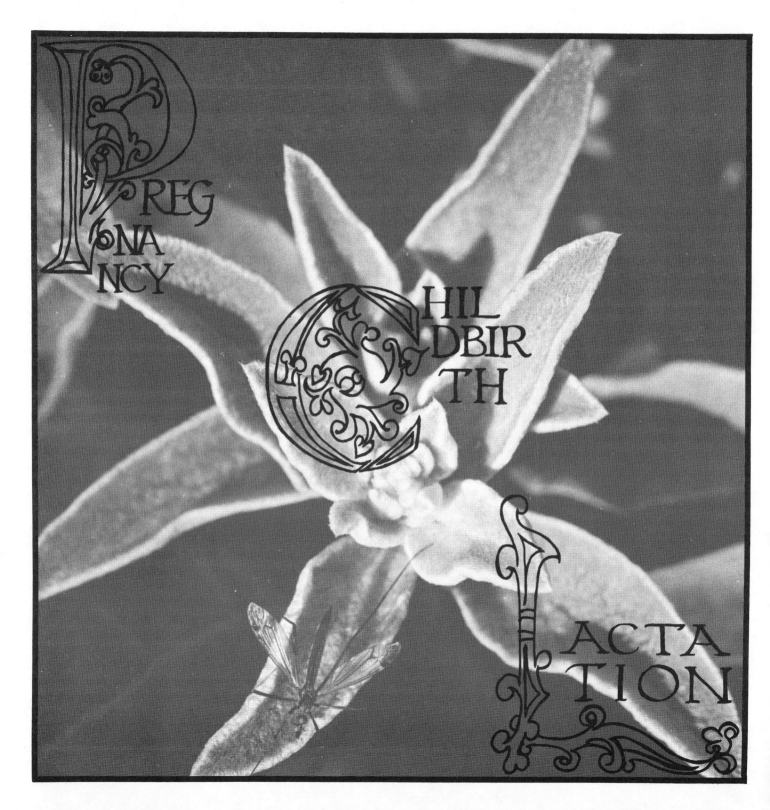

PREGNANCY

CHILDBIRTH

LACTATION

Pregnancy, Childbirth & Lactation Herbs

Angelica *Archangelica officinalis. Umbelliferae. See Emenogues.*

Balm *Melissa officinales. Labiatae. See "Infertility".*

Bayberry *Myrica cerfica "myrtle". "American vegetable". Specific for the ovaries and womb troubles, douche. A valuable check for profuse menstruation and especially is unfailing when combined with Shepherds Purse. The tree is an emblem of love and it's said Venus herself used myrtle as a douche or skin wash to be more seductive.*

Cayenne *Capsicum. Useful for juandice. Very good in leukorrhea and generally has excellent effects on the female organs. The influence is most beneficial on the womb in pregnancy.*

Beth Root. *Trillium pendulum. "Birth Root", "Milk Ipeacac", "Lamb's Quarters", "Jew's Harp Plant", "Three leaved Nightshade". Used for excessive menses, leucorrhea, lax conditions of the vagina and fallen womb. For all womb troubles, female complaints.*

Betony *See Wood Betony*

Birthwort *Arisolchia clematitis, Aristolochiaceae. This herb is included as a metaphorical aid to understand the relationship of snake symbology and sex. A drop of the juice of Birthwort will kill any snake and the people who cover themselves with this juice make themselves immune to snakebite. Used formerly following birth for bloody discharge. The name Aristoslochiacea means "Best Birth". Its acid strengthens the function of leucocytes in resisting infection.*

Bisort Root *Polygonum bistorta. "Patience Dock", "Dragonworth", "Snake Weed", "Easter Grant". Excellent for leukorrhea. When combined with plantain, used for gonorrhea. Used as a douche to decrease or regulate the menstrual flow.*

Black Western Choke Cherry *Prunus serotina ehrh. The Arakara used the berry juice for pain during childbirth. Also called "Black Cherry" and used to treat muscular soreness.*

120

Blessed Thistle   *Cnicus benedictus. See "Temporary Sterility".*

Borage   *Borago officinalis. Arab women eat the leaves and flowers in salads: so do I. The seeds and leaves are wonderful for nursing mothers; contains much potassium and will increase the milk supply. Used for sore hearts, literally, and metaphorically as it strengthens hearts and dispels "melancholy or heart-sickness". This herb is easy to grow and once established, may take over your garden. The bluish, pentacle-shaped flowers are a delight to bees.*

Buckwheat   *Hopi Indians used an infusion of the whole plant to relieve pain in childbirth. The "wild buckwheat" or "painted cup" (See Indian paintbrush) was also used as menstrual medicine .*

Burdock   *Arctium lappa compositae. It works specifically on the ovaries. Kloss. Found on waste places and roadsides and often disliked by sheep farmers as a pastureweed for it's tenacity on to wool. "Good for nothing", the farmer said, "as he made a sweep at the burdock's head." Decrease the value of his wool crop. May be used externally for swellings caused by syphilis. Add Burdock to the wash water before cleaning, and it is also reported to purify a room.*

Carrot   *See Wild Carrot.*

Caraway   *Carum carvi. "Common Caraway". Stomach and uterine cramps are obviated. It promotes milk building in nursing mothers to keep a baby or child healthy, free from illness (or evil spirits). Sew some seeds into a small bag and tuck it under the mattress where the child sleeps.*

Capsicum   *See Cayenne.*

Catnip   *Nepeta cataria L. See "Emmenagogues".*

Cayenne   *Capsicum. See "Infertility".*

Chamomile   *Matricaria Chomilla. See "Emmenagogues".*

Comfrey   *Symphytum officinalis. See "Anaphrodisiacs".*

Cornflower   *Centaura cyanis compositae. "Bachelor's Buttons". Folk remedy for leukorrhea. A few flowers can be eaten raw in salads. Also make a tea of the flowers and take a cup two times daily. Action improved with the addition of aromatic herbs such as rosemary, thyme, etc.*

Cornsmut   *Ustilago Zene. Actually, a fungus used by the Zuni to hasten childbirth by increasing the severity* of labor. Also, given for postpartum hemorrhage. A pinch in a small quantity of warm or cold water and taken at intervals.

Cotton Root   See "Emmenagogues".

Cramp Bark   Viburnum opulus. The flowers and leaves are called prunifolium or black-haw or American Sloe. Has been recommended in abortions. The active principle is Viburnim and is used in a dose of 5 - 6 grams. Hermann. It relaxes spasms and relieves cramps. Muhr.*Also, one of the "Estrogen Balancers" in herbal remedy as a menstrual corrective. A decoction of the twigs is used to treat uterine pains and the bark for hemorrhage of the womb. Also, called "highbrush cranberry" and used to treat uterine infections and septic poisonings following childbirth.

Creeping Thyme & Thyme   Thymus seryphilum labiatae. The "women's herb" of central Europe and the Alps in folk medicine. Excellent taken hot for suppressed or obstructed menses. Thymus vulgaris will produce perspiration when taken hot. Also, called "Mother of Thyme". This herb was given, in folk medicine, in the Alps, to pregnant women. Good bath for sickly children.

Cubeb Berries   See "Aphrodisiacs".

Dandelion Root   Taraxicum dens-leonis or Taratanum officinalis. Compositae. "Puff-Ball", "White Endive", "Priest's Crown". Dandelion has 28 parts sodium. The natural nutritive salts purify the blood and destroy the acids in the blood. Good for anemia. Has a beneficial effect upon the female organs. Kloss. Helps in diabetes, obesity and over-sleepiness. Excellent for general female troubles. A. Riva writes if you bury the dandelion under the northwest corner of the house, it will bring favorable winds to the property and its inhabitants. Also as a bath herb, it aids those of us with psychic talents, or siddhis, to summon spirits when necessary. The Irish called it "heart-fever-grass" and it purifies the blood and overcomes despondency.

Devil's Bit Scabious   Scabiosa succisa. Dip sacaceae. Strongly honey-scented flowers. Legend says that this plant is so beneficial to humans that the devil bit a piece off the root hoping to kill the plant. Especially good for female disorders, vaginitis, menstrual irregularity, uterine disorders, also venereal disease. Make a brew of the flowers. Also a nervine.

Double Tansy   See Tansy.

Echinacea   See "Aphrodisiacs".

Erigeron   Powa wi. Used by Hopi as a menstruation medicine, but also by Hopi to expedite childbirth. Alfred Whiting's **Ethnobotany of the Hopis,** Bulletin No. 15, Museum of Arizona. Also called "desert trumpet" and "wild buckwheat".

*See page 33

False Solomon's Seal   *Smilacina stellata. See Permanent Sterility.*

Fennel   *Foeniculum officinale. Umbelliferae. Will relieve jaundice. The foliage improves memory and is a tonic for the brain. Roots, a laxative, good for womb troubles. The leaves or seeds are boiled in barley water and drunk by lactating women to increase their supply and make it more wholesome. Contains sulphur, potassium and organic sodium. Other flowers like marigold don't seem to grow very well around fennel, I've noticed. Use fennel for bloating before or during menstruation and if needed, at midcycle (ovulation). It's from too much estrogen (or possibly too much fluid intake).*

Feverfew   *Matricaria parthenium. Compositae. Very helpful in preventing miscarriage and to aid in a difficult labor or retention of afterbirth. Used also for female hysteria and infertility. Levy. Chrysanthemum parthenium or Pyrethrum parthenium. Large quantities simmered in water for bathing of the genitals. Used in the 18th century as a tea for female hysteria, to strengthen the womb and even then known to expel the placenta and enable women to conceive. Rose. The dried flowers have been said to be abortifacients.*

Filaree   *Alfierilla spp. "Storksbill", "Pinklets". Excellent for pregnancy. Reported to increase the milk supply of any mammal. To treat for gonorrhea, take equal amounts of yerba del burro (distuchlis spicata) and filaree, sweeten and take simmered in the morning and night for awhile. J. Rose.*

Flax   *See Yellow Flax.*

Garden Mercury   *Mercurialis annua. Hippocrates had it applied to the sexual parts to expel the placenta.*

Garlic   *Allium sativum Lilicaen. See "Aphrodisiacs".*

Golden Seal   *Hydrastis canadinsis. "Yellow Puccoon". Use the root. "Taken in small but frequent doses, it will allay nausea in pregnancy. Steep a tsp. in a pint of boiling water for 20 minutes, stir and let settle. Pour off tea and take 6 tbsp. a day." Kloss. I have read NOT to take Golden Seal when pregnant in large doses, or not at all. One of the Cherokee's favorite plants. Used as a douche in treatment of leukorrhea, especially combined with myrrh. I had a friend who, becoming pregnant,* **while nursing her son just over one year,** *decided to wean her child. He didn't take to this turn of events at all and was very persistent in efforts to nurse. She then applied golden seal to her nipples to dissuade him by its startling taste. He seemed to like it, and continued for some length of time.*

Hardhack   *Spiraea tomentosa L. "Whitecap", "Silverweed". A tea made from the flowers and leaves has been used during pregnancy and to ease child birth.*

Holy Thistle   *See "Temporary Sterility".*

Hops   *Humul lupus. Urticacea. See "Anaphrodiacs".*

Juniper   *(Common). Juniperus communis L. See "Temporary Sterility".*

Lady's Fern   *Washington Indians used a tea of the boiled stems to stop postpartum hemorrhage. Linked with the maiden hair fern, who when placed under water takes on a silvery appearance, yet remains dry. The ancients claimed her to be the hair of Venus - after Aphrodite, who rose from the sea. The Romans attributed the Graces, Beauty and Love, to this herb.*

Lady's Mantle   *Alchemilla vulgaris. Rosaceae. See "Infertility".*

Lavendar   *Lavendula spica and Lavendula vera. Labiatae. See Emmenagogues".*

Licorice Root   *Glycyrrhiza lipidota. Nytt. See "Infertility".*

Marigold   *Calendula officinalis. See "Emmenagogues".*

Marijuana   *See "Herbs for the Mind".*

Milkwort   *Polygala vulgaris. Polygalaceae and Polygala amarella. Used to increase the milk supply of nursing women. Named from the Greek, "gala" meaning much milk. It also cools the blood. Eat a handful, raw, twice daily.*

Mint   *Mentha spicata. See "Emmenagogues".*

Mistletoe   *Pharadendron flavescens. A weak tea was given to regulate contractions if the mother was having a hard time during labor among the Wiyots of N. California. Vogel cites the use of this herb as a contraceptive also.*

Mugwort   *Artemisia vulgaris. See "Emmenagogues".*

Myrtle   *See Bayberry bark. Married couples in Roman times of festivity always wore wreaths of myrtle towards preserving Youth and Love. The herb was also associated with Hymen, son of Venus and symbol of "unchaste love". Bridegrooms would wear it as a headress in Roman times also. One tradition has it that a dream of Myrtle portended a second marriage, if the dreamer was already betrothed. · If not, it indicated a numerous family, wealth and healthy old age.*

Nettle   *Urtica dioica. "Common Stinging Nettle". This herb can be used as an astringent for hemorrhage* of the womb. It contains a lot of iron. *Jeanne Rose*. Juliette de Baircle-Levy says it's the "white" or "blind" nettle, *lamium album. Labiatae* which stems bleeding from the womb and over heavy menses, as a douche and as local applications, soaked on cloth. *Kloss* adds it increases the menstrual flow.

Oatstraw *Avena sativa. Gramineae.* Low in starch, high in mineral content (especially phosphorus and potassium and magnesium and calcium, highly bone building and nerve tonic so great for pregnancy, lactation). Useful in a tea taking equal parts of mugwort, cramp bark and chamomile for menstrual cramps.

Orchis *Orchis maculata.* See "Infertility".

Painted Cup *Castilleja linariae folia.* "Indian Paintbrush" A Hopi menstrual medicine.

Palebeard Tongue *Penstemon pallidus small.* Another metaphorical herb. The root has been used to treat rattlesnake bites and to hasten the movement of the afterbirth in a newly delivered woman.

Papoose Root See Blue Cohosh.

Peach Leaves *Prunus persica.* Used as a specific for ailing ovaries. Also, for womb troubles and burning itching genitals. *Kloss.* The fruit is rich in Vitamin A and little protein and fat and contains less calories than apples or pears. But bear in mind the image of the man-bred peach tree, so heavy with huge fruit propped up by our desires for bigger and juicier peaches. Small is beautiful as Schumacher writes, and better for us nutritionally. It is also used for treating morning sickness in pregnant women.

Peppermint See Mint.

Periwinkle *Vinca major and minor. Apocynacea.* Checks hemorrhage from the vagina. It's used to control over abundant milk and to dry up milk when weaning. However, ideal weaning happens so gradually neither herbs or other solutions are needed to help this process. No one can enter a house with periwinkle hanging on the door. Wards off evil spirits. For trichomonas infections, a douche of chapperal with slippery elm, oatstraw and periwinkle is helpful. If you are congested or bloated with a late period, try drinking periwinkle with motherwort.

Piperita *Menth piperita. Labiatae.* "Balm Mint". Great warming qualities. Stops vomiting, is anti-bacterial. Good for gas pains. Also for painful menstruation. It's a general tonic for the whole body and a specific remedy for a headache. Take several hot cups and soak feet in a peppermint bath. Use the pulp for swelling breasts. Dioscorides claimed that mint was an aphrodisiac.

Plantain *Plantago major.* Women from the Middle Ages have used Plantain for all female complaints.

"It is thought to cure the head of antipathy to Mars and to cure the private parts by sympathy to Venus". Jeanne Rose. A decoction of the leaves with Myrtle for a douche. Drink daily, it's reported to promote fertility. The Indians used it, whole plant. Use internally and externally for syphyllis. Plantain is a favorite of mine and I always seem to have a front yard full of these dark green beauties. "Stays all manners of flowing, even women's courses, when too abundant", Kloss.

Raspberry

Rubus idaeus. Rosaceae. See "Infertility".

Red Clover

Trifolium pratense. Leguminosae. See "Infertility".

Rosemary Leaves

Rosmarinus officinalis. Labiatae.

The Gypsies love this herb that beautifies women. The Arabs sprinkle the dried powdered herb on the umbilicus of a new-born. It's an astringent and antiseptic. Good for nursing mothers. The babies will receive it through the milk. The gypsies hang sprigs in their vans as protection against evil forces, especially by sleeping infants and children. Rosemary was put into wedding bouquets. There was a saying in Europe that wherever Rosemary flourished in a garden, the master in the house was female. Drinking Rosemary water is said to do away with all body evil; however, excessive doses can be fatal. Kloss lists it with cures for "female trouble". My dear herbalist friend, Rosemary Gladstar, gives this name greater meaning.

Safflower

Carthamus tinctorius. Compositae. Used to treat irregular menstruation and a gentle laxative.

Saffron

To increase the menstrual flow. Kloss. Irish women are said to dye their robes with saffron to give their limbs strength. Also worn by Swamis in India.

Sandalwood

This herb, native to India, is used by women in pregnancy who are freaking out. The wind called ANANT VAYU, which enters a woman with child through the soles of her feet, is responsible for the emotional lability of pregnancy. Lability, not liability, for having one's feelings moved freely through your being is a great "side-effect" of increased progesterone during pregnancy, and ovulation for that matter. Sandalwood, applied as a paste between one's toes, grounds the woman, helping her to balance between pleasure and pain.

We are all familiar with this as an incense. Yet in the Burman Empire, on the last day of the year (April 12th) the women mixed sandlewood with rose water and sprinkled it on all whom they met to symbolize the washing away of impurities of the old year and the starting of the new, without sin. According to legend, King Solomon's temples were built of this wood, and carrying a chip of it was considered a very lucky amulet.

Sarsaparilla

Smilax aristolochiaefolia or officinalis. Pirates used this herb as a remedy for syphillis. "One of the best herbs to use for infants infected with V.D." Kloss. The juices of the plant given to a newborn, as legend has it, makes the little one immune from poisons". Also, called "Jamaica", "Quay-Quill", "Red Sarsaparilla". Sassafras is usually mixed with it to act as a synergistic. However, in Dr. Christopher's Female Corrective, Sarsaparilla is included without sassafras. Riva says the dried root prolongs life, excites the passions, causing men to be more virile and women to be more sensual. It also hinders premature aging.

Saw Palmetto Berries

Serenoa serulata or *Serpens*. See "Aphrodisiacs".

Sheperd's Purse

Capsella bursa pastoris. "Cocowort", "St. James Weed", "Shepherd's Heary". Has a rhythmic impulse upon the sexual region of women and will decrease the menstrual flow. After birthing twins, I began to hemorrhage. My Shepherd's Purse was brewed with bayberry bark in a matter of minutes. I drank the warmed tea, replacing fluids and stopping the frightening blood flow. It contains much vitamin K, the blood clotting element, and vitamin C. She is used as a pot herb for the kitchen in Europe and during olden days - and is still used today. Used in the Far East as a delicious addition to a salad. In India, it's often used and tastes somewhat like cabbage. The seed pods resemble a heart in shape. It's also called "Mother's Heart".

Slippery Elm Bark

Ulmus fulva. I've used this as a soothing paste on an itching and burning cunt. Just mix a little water with the powder to a smooth consistency. Used as an enema for babies with inflamed bowels and as a vaginal douche for women. It's an excellent nutritive food for children as well. Good for womb troubles. As a douche for leukorrhea, and general female discomforts. Riva says that wearing Slippery Elm in a small flannel bag and hanging it on a thong about the neck will encourage a person to be good in speech and language. In any case, she is a well-known lozenge for sore throats.

Smooth Upland Sumac

Rhus glabrum. "Smooth Sumac". Omahas boiled fruits and applied externally as a liquid wash for pain in childbirth. Useful for gonorrhea and syphyllis, equal parts sumac berries and bark, white pine bark and slippery elm. Valuable for leukorrhea also.

Spearmint

See Mint.

Spikenard

Aralia racemosa. Use the root to make childbirth easy and speedy. Take the tea for quite some time before labor begins. With equal parts of **Spikenard**, Wintergreen and Sassafras for treating V.D. Kloss. Dr. Christopher includes this herb in his "Change-ease" formula to be given one month for every year of damage, six days on, 1 day off.

Sprouts

YOU DO IT! Use any seed. Be it herbal or vegetable. Reported to be aphrodisiacs, sprouts will increase vitality. When pregnant or considering conception, sprouting seeds and tending them is an excellent activity. It's metaphorically valuable, as well as nutritious, for both you and baby. My children, from conception on, have loved sprouts, ideal "finger food". It's nature's healer along with chlorophyll, wheatgrass, comfrey, and alfalfa. All you need is a canning jar and rim, strong nylon netting,(sold in hardware stores as screening) seeds, water, and daily attention. Experiment around with various lengths of soaking for different seeds and how often to rinse. Eat when you hear them call out to you in perfect juiciness and vivaciousness. Read Kulvinkas's work on sprouts.

127

Squaw Vine   *Mitchella repens. "Partridge Berry", "Winter Clover", "Hive Vine", "Deer Berry". Make sure you don't get "Squaw tea" instead, or also knowns as "Mormon tea" which resembles sticks and branches. Squawvine is leafy and much more expensive. Increases menstrual flow. Helpful for leukorrhea and womb troubles. Kloss. This was my favorite pregnancy herb, combined with raspberry. Always had a chilled jar in the refrigerator on hot days and sun warm tea on the mellow days of late pregnancy.*

St. John's Wort   *Hypericum perforatum. Very good for chronic uterine troubles, after pain in childbirth and is said to correct irregular menstruation. Good in hysteria and as a fomentation and ointment for caked breast. Will increase menstrual flow. Kloss.*

Storksbill   *See Filaree.*

Sundew   *Droser rotundifolia. Droseraceae. For morning sickness in pregnant women.*

Tansy   *Tanacetum vulgare L. See "Emmenagogues".*

Thyme   *Thymus vulgaris. See "Emmenagogues".*

Water Pepper   *Polygonum punctatum. See "Emmenagogues".*

White Oak Bark   *Querous alba. See "Anaphrodisiacs".*

Wild Cherry   *Prunus virginiana. "Common Chokecherry". Cherokees used this herb to relieve pain in childbirth. Use the inner bark, as an infusion. Chokecherry juice (p. melanocarpo) was given to drink in case of post partum hemorrhage. Pits of cherries contain cyanide and could cause death. Cooking the fruit frees the poison, the sourness will disappear.*

Wild Ginger   *Asarum Canadense. Zingiberaceae. Used as a contraceptive boiled slowly in a small amount of water for a long time. The root is not actually "wild" but imported from China and West Africa. Good for delayed menstruation and for exhaustion following child birth. Also helpful, as a warm drink for childbirth pains, especially with honey and lemon. It will increase the menstrual flow. Chewed, it's an immediate remedy for menstrual cramps.*

128

Wild Yam *Dioscorea villosa. "Colic Root", "China Root", "Devils Bones". One of the best herbs for general pain in pregnancy, taken during whole time. Very relaxing and soothing to the nerves. Will allay morning sickness in small doses and combined with ginger, helps prevent miscarriages. Good with squawvine in later part of pregnancy Steep a heaping tsp. in a cup of boiling water 30 minutes. Drink cold 1 - 3 cups daily. The root of the Wild Yam in Mexico and Central America contains the synthesis of the complex steroids which eventually go into making the "Pill". It was also used by the Meskwaki and Chippewa Indians as a decoction to relieve labor pains.*

Witch Hazel *Hamamelis virginica. Unsurpassed for stopping excessive menstruation. Internally, steep a heaping tsp. in a cup of boiling water 30 minutes. Take one or more cupsful during the day as needed, a large mouthful at a time, says Kloss. The shoots have been used for hundreds of years as divining rods for water.*

Wood Betony *Betonica officinalis L. "Betony". Culpepper says "This herb is appropriated to the planet Jupiter and the sign Aries and causes an easy and speedy delivery of women in childbirth". Ancient dreamers said Betony would protect the dreamer from monsters and other scary visions and dreams. A good preventative for witchcraft. Used also to decrease the menstrual flow. Sprinkle inside the home near doorway and windows. Riva writes that Betony forms a protective wall against evil spirits and witches.*

Wood Sanicle *See Sanicle.*

Wuta'Kvala *Tetradymia canescens inermis. A decoction of this plant has been given to a laboring woman if her uterus fails to contract properly. Hopi medicinal herb, a low gray shrub with yellow flowers.*

Yellow Flax *Linum astrale. Hopi women used this internally and externallly in cases of protracted labor. This herb is known as "weasel medicine" because the "weasel when in danger of being captured, rapidly digs its way thru the ground and comes out another place." So the herb encourages the baby thru the birth canal, says Whiting. Riva reports flax, kept in the home, protects from disturbing outside influences and promotes peacefulness within. And a child running through a field of flax or carrying some around on their person, is said to become very beautiful.*

Zinc *See "Infertility".*

Dear Jeannine Parvati,

Thank you very much for helping me with the information you gave me when I visited with you. I really enjoyed reading the information on birth control and conscious dreaming.

I wanted to ask you if you were going to mention the Indian's use of False Hellebore in your new book. I saw False Hellebore mentioned in Jeanne Rose's book and in your handout. I got really freaked out to think of anyone possibly using this herb if there was any chance of pregnancy (first trimester). If sheep feed on this plant (Veratrum Californicum) during the second or third weeks after conception, many of the offspring are cycloptic (one eye) and most have severe cronical malformations. It apparently affects the transfer RNA in the fetus in some way and the facial skeletal structure doesn't develop normally. Now, the sheep are eating the folliage and the Indians use cured root, but the idea of severely deformed babies makes me wish there was some way to warn women of the potential hazards associated with this plant. A more complete description is in Kingsbury's **POISONOUS PLANTS OF THE UNITED STATES**. Kingsbury sometimes calls plants poisonous on fairly flimsy evidence, but the case against False Hellebore is fairly well documented.

I was interested in attending the class (X) on November 18, about starting non-profit educational corporation etc. Please let me know if it would be okay to come for one class and how much the fee would be.

I am looking forward to seeing your new book in print. I hope it comes out soon.

Thanks again for your help,
Ann

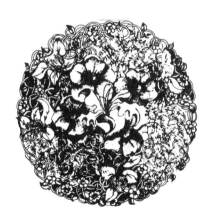

Celestial Influences

"It is important to rightly picture the condition of pregnancy. The soul and spirit of the woman are to a certain extent displaced from her physical body, and she becomes thereby more connected with the heavens (spacey, I call it); the child, on the other hand, is descending from the spiritual world and gradually shaping its earthly body." pg. 13

"The great connection that exists between the stars and the developing embryo has already been mentioned. In considering the human form, we must take into account the relationship between the forming of the head, chest, and limbs on the one hand, and the constellations of the zodiac on the other. In ancient times when people were familiar with such knowledge, this relationship was expressed by writing the sign of the Ram against the forehead, and the sign of the Fishes against the feet. The whole being of (wo)man was thus fitted into those twelve constellations of the zodiac through which circle the sun, moon and planets. It makes a great difference whether the influence of the stars is experienced from within the mother or from outside her. Before birth, the forces of the stars work on the form of the child when it is surrounded by the embryonic membranes and the mother's body. After birth, having cast off its covering, the newborn baby is exposed directly to these forces. This moment of birth is one of great importance for the child. It is a completely new situation, like the change from a bud to a blossom. Something new is created.

It is important to know that the individual, in coming down to the parents, strives to be born under a constellation he has already chosen.

In our times, many people will consider such a statement fantastic. Great personalities, however, have been concerned with the stellar influences. It is impressive to read Goethe's ideas about his own birth constellation. It is quite clear that Goethe waited for the hour of the constellation under which he wanted to enter this world.

How much one would like to recommend to the modern obstetrician to give heed to such thoughts. Science and medicine have forgotten to give heed to such thoughts. It is to be wished that scientists and doctors might have more veneration for the occurances of nature than many show at present. From the point of view from which this book is conceived, no attempt should ever be made to speed up a birth unless it is absolutely necessary for medical reasons. Disturbances will be brought into the life of the individual if he is born at a time other than the chosen one." page 20. by Norbert Glas, M.D.

CONCEPTION, BIRTH & EARLY CHILDHOOD, Anthroposophic Press, Inc. 258 Hollow Road, Spring Valley, New York 10977

I would like to add that the words in parentheses are mine. And that using herbs to speed up or slow down labor unless absolutely necessary is also disturbing. Rarely do we need the help of herbs in birthing. Usually we can work out the problem via touch, counseling and channeling. As birthing is a passage for souls, psychological approaches are extremely helpful. Of course it can be argued that any time of birth is the right one. The moment that is meant to be or else it would not have happened. Yet we can respect natural rhythms, or with impatience interfere. Herbs can be used with either intention. Choose wisely.

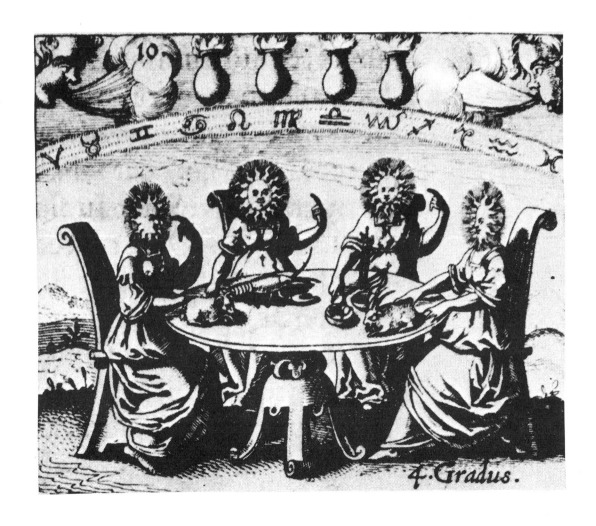

Dear Jeannine (Parvati),

With three children already here on earth with us (and a new embryo presently developing!). I have been blessed with diverse experiences in sexuality, conception, birth, and natural birth control. The subject at hand is natural birth control, and it seems natural to discuss my encounters chronologically.

My first son, Siddhartha, was born in 1969, at a time when there was a relative dearth of enlightened information on childbirth and natural birth control. Unfortunately, he was not granted a prepared homebirth and long-term breastfeeding as his siblings were to later experience. After he was born, I was "talked into" an I.U.D. by hospital personnel. I never felt really "right" about it; it was the first and last technological birth control device I was ever to use. (I could never convince myself to take "the Pill" - my intuition forbade it!). Within a few months, my husband and I began meditational/devotional practices. In one of my Master's books, I read of the subtle psychic effects of birth control on women. Yes, the effects were unfavorable, and interfered with spiritual progress. But at that time, our family planning problem took care of itself; out came the I.U.D. for we had decided upon a celibate discipline (for awhile) to aid in our spiritual undertakings. When the cosmic urge for the conception of another child came upon us, the temporary celibacy came to a close. (We never used that method again, incidentally!)

Shanti, the second son, was born in 1971. The family's first home birth! After his birth, I depended wholly upon breastfeeding/ total mothering, as my protection against conception. I was one of the fortunate women whose feminine processes remained suspended in amenorrhea for 18 months. Natural child-spacing can be a reality, I discovered. During the ovulation after my first period, I happened to become pregnant again.

Perhaps I had grown more aware of the mother-birth processes of the universe, for I was more attuned to them. Near the time of this third conception, I was visited on the other planes by a loving, feminine soul, in a dream. She indicated that I would be pregnant by gesturing to my womb. This being reminded me so much of a traditional Catholic saint, that we named our first daughter Clare, after St. Clare of Assisi.

After Clare was born in the Christmas season of 1973, I experienced amenorrhea for 2 years. Even better than before! However, I had read in the Ostrander/Schroeder book, **Natural Birth Control**, that intercourse during the astrologically fertile period could possibly result in a pregnancy even while the mother was breast-feeding and not menstruating. So, I had the appropriate charts made and we abstained from making love on those few, four days a month - as an added insurance! Then I began investigating other forms of natural family planning as information was released. When my cycles resumed this time, I had decided to combine astrological birth control with the ovulation method of detecting the changes in cervical mucous.

I think it is absolutely essential, now that I have made the discovery myself, that every woman should be aware of her personal, unique cycles and her body's individual signals. Not only did I realize my ovulation each month, but I could reconcile emotional patterns and manifestations of libido to their natural courses. It had seemed like such an incomprehensible jumble before! And this "awareness" worked perfectly for about six months; the only disadvantage being the occasional irritability of my husband on the days of abstinence! We were becoming more in tune with my rhythms when our Karma changed toward conception again.

This past May, during the time I positively detected as my monthly ovulation, I had another dream experience, similar in its intensity to that of Clare's. And in this dream, I met a wonderful male figure whom I felt I had always known. I did not know how I could express my spiritual love for him. I felt intensely loving after this time, and extremely desirous of making love, even though I knew conception was likely that week. Needless to say, I am carrying my fourth child!

While my husband and I have used celibacy, breastfeeding, complete mothering, and astrological/ovulation methods of natural family planning, we have also tried to remain receptive to extra-terrestial, spiritual signals that indicate a soul has chosen us to prepare a physical vehicle for him/her. Perhaps we plan these family matters, or are aware of our inter-relating karma, before any of us take human birth. And in our veil of forgetfulness, we need extraordinary reminders that we are to be rejoined by still another dear one, whom we had temporarily forgotten. But in the meantimes, between such births, it is wise to employ harmless and natural systems of birth control until these messages come through.

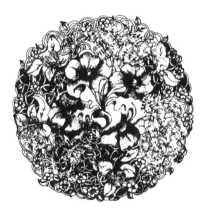

Karen

The Menopause ⁕ the Change

*T*HE CHANGE - *A time in women's lives to be celebrated, not endured. But how is this possible when our health is failing? Some writers[1], seeing the monthly bleedings as opportunities for elimination of toxins in the system, are convinced that the uncomfortable symptoms of menopause are due to the cessation of this purification. In other words, once bleeding stops, the organism is backed up with impurities. Hence the headaches, rapid loss of sexual interest,[2] irritability, backache, menopausal arthritus, and many other disease conditions become manifest. It is a sad commentary on our general state of health. What we, as young women, can do now, in preparation for this very important **rite of passage**[3], is to consciously aim our health building practices to include the herbs for women's health. We will then be including many estrogen containing foods in plant forms and later, not need the synthetic estrogens the medical industry offers. First and foremost, a healthy **attitude**, or positive thought forms, about menopause is in order. Welcoming this process as a natural one, without regret for the cessation of fertility, will go a long way toward remedying our culture's current approach to "the Change". Presently, most women who can afford it, rush off to their doctors at the first "hot flash" for synthetic estrogen or Premarin (not that much better than "synthetic" estrogen). By taking these drugs, symptoms are relieved, but the incidence of cancer, blood clots, and heart disease has been shown greatly to be increased.[4]*

*The understandable hunt for the fountain of youth; menopause reminds us we are indeed mortal, and now unable to reproduce ourselves. The most secure feminist must pause at this time, too - and re-examine what is important for the remainder of her time here on Earth. If what is important is impinged upon by poor health, now is the time to correct this. No more can we pollute our bodies through the American diet, with its insane emphasis on high protein intake and "pleasure", valueless foods. Each and every substance taken in most likely will become our very **being**; never again will our excesses and harmful materials be eliminated monthly through the menstrual flow. This is it, folks. Now, what if the menstruation **isn't** an act of elimination. Our fail-safe mechanism to insure the best health for potential off spring? Does this cancel out what you've just read? It proves an interesting way to live, if nothing else, to imagine that each and every substance you ingest becomes **you** - the basic, material you, as well as your thoughts, feelings, and how you relate with the world. But this is another story - how **diet** affects us as women; the way we perceive our female processes, and how well we can love ourselves.*

*And so the remaining portion of this chapter is devoted to our menopausal sisters - in the knowledge that with rightful health practices and some cultural support, the "Change" may be experienced as a liberation - ah! At last a crone,[5] freed from the **obvious** nature of being female. Our opportunity to focus energy into the more subtle aspects of being a woman, as the natural process of menopause unfolds within us.*

What appears most important during menopause is the adequate supply of trace-minerals, and minerals

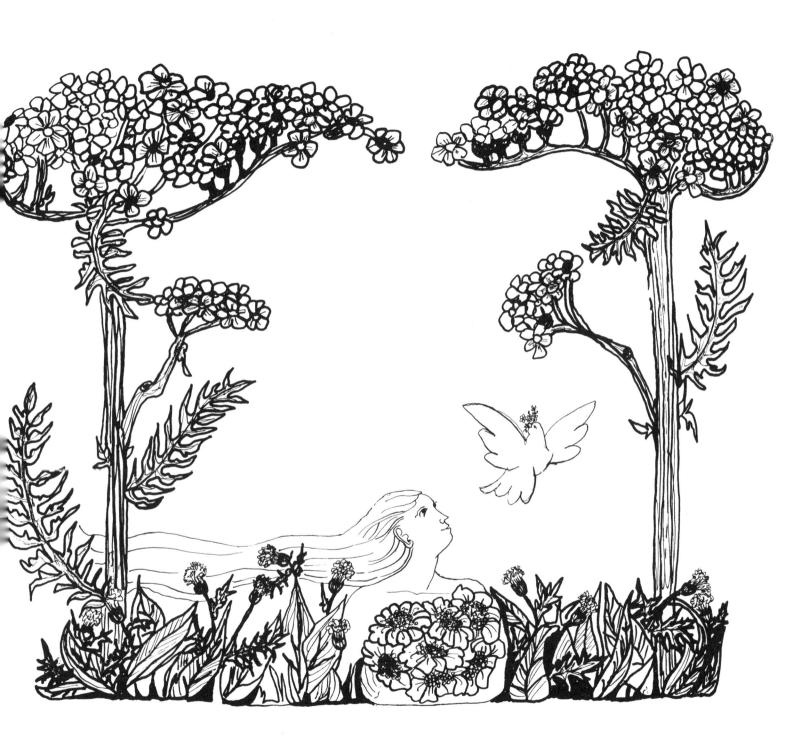

as catalysts for *enzyme functions*. Then, the usual course of hormone production during menopause is shifted to the adrenal glands from the ovaries, who now retire[5A]. And a well deserved rest it is! Each newborn female has within her ovaries all the eggs she'll need during a lifetime - not only do the ovaries cyclically release these eggs, or ova, but also produce progesterone during the lutein phase, or mid-cycle. During pregnancy, the ovaries also produce progesterone for awhile until the placenta takes over this function. But when the adrenals are exhausted due to poor nutrition, repressed rage, and improper liver functioning, the organism is in need of additional estrogen. I'm aware this is an over-simplification of a very involved process. Again, I am writing not from personal experience, either. Yet I do see that my sisters who eat in "unconventional", or **health-conscious** ways, experience their menopause as no big deal, whereas, those of us who ignore the signals our bodies give about proper diet and attitude toward menstruation, experience the menopause as agony. Perhaps by understanding somewhat the serious effects that synthetic estrogen has on us, we will awaken to a more natural, simple diet using herbs.

Synthetic estrogen increases the need for vitamin E - the element so vital for proper sexual functioning. Premarin, billed as a "natural" form of estrogen, (supposedly, one might think it's considered more "organic" because it's collected from the urine of mares, and we all know that horses are "natural") potentially causes the dangerous blood-clots - same as the synthetic kinds.[6]

The human body is an ecology system too. We know what happens when man-made chemicals are indiscriminately added to our natural resources. Using synthetic estrogen is bad ecology. If you, as reader, are now taking estrogen by injection or pill, I refer you to Dr. Paavo Airola's work on this subject. And to the following list of herbs used by women to aid them during the "Change". Hormones, i.e. sex hormones, are made up from the foods and herbs we ingest. There are many hormone precursors. Foods and herbs that stimulate or are vital in the production of your natural hormones. When a woman comes off synthetic estrogen, she may be alarmed to experience rapid aging. Some herbs are suggested with this in mind. Many have the reputation for slowing down the aging process. Yet, it is regular attention to diet, rest, love, and spiritual practice (sadhana) that really slows lows down the aging process. Many **yoga** practices (pranyamas, and asanas) are reported to reverse aging. I know one beautiful example of this. An herbalist who at 80 looks 50, who attributes this to her usage of herbs, careful nutrition, and her ability to use "air as food". She practices regular pranyamas and says these breath controlling exercises are a meal in itself. A love for children and ability to enter a "baby space" also has this effect. In any case, not only do food and herbs act like hormone precursors in my mind, but spirit does as well. Let us begin with how we may best nourish ourselves in our golden years. Here is a beginning list of herbs useful for menopause:

Mexican Wild Yam, Sassafras, Licorice (Aletris Farinosa), **Lady's Slipper, Life Root, Passion Flower, Black Cohosh, Honduras Sarasparilla, False Unicorn Root** (Helonias Dioica), **Elder.** These all contain some natural estrogen which can help even after a hysterectomy.

And some foods: (By no means a complete list.)

Seeds, Sprouts, Whole grains, Royal Jelly, Bee Pollen, Bananas.

One nutritionist[7] writes that cholesterol is needed by our bodies as the matrix for all hormones and this is why fertile eggs are known to "enhance libido". She recommends the use of tiny amounts of dairy (please make it goat - cows are just too big!) which is unprocessed, or raw (yogurt is fine.).

Stan Malstrom recommends the following herbal recipe for menopause:[8]

Blessed Thistle, Squaw Vine, Raspberry Leaves, Golden Seal, Lobelia, Gravelroot, Ginger Root, Cayenne, Parsley and Marshmallow Root. There are many formulas also marketed. Dr. Christopher's "Change-Ease" for example. These are sold in capsules and you can swallow them or let the powdered herbs dissolve into a cup of tea. Remember to take them on an empty stomach for remedial purposes.

Raymond Dextreit, in his wonderful book, **Our Earth, Our Cure**, noted that if menopause occurs after the age of fifty, it's a much easier process. Going so far to say that it *should* occur after fifty, is missing the point, however. He adds that if there's a fibroid tumor present in the uterus, menopause will be postponed. My hope is to let this measuring, or quantifying of women's experiences onto some linear time table, fall by the wayside. Menopause, the cessation of ovulation and menstruation, comes at the perfect time for each woman's experience of her own sexuality - *whenever* that is. He goes on to share some important suggestions. That foods from the vegetable kingdom, including herbs, best favor the glandular functions and relieve congestion, strengthening the nervous system. So often there is a rising of copper while using the synthetic estrogen - causing emotional instability, and a decrease of zinc, causing depression. Herbs help to bring these trace minerals back into balance. He advises us to completely eliminate meat, sugar, coffee, alcohol and any chemical type of food (many nutritionists agree on this) and limit animal foods to occassional eggs & buttermilk. Lemon, as well as garlic and parsley, are excellent for this time. So are the culinary herbs which stimulate the circulation. So often "hot flashes", dizziness, perspiration are the signal that you are congested and these herbs help relieve this problem: **Chervil, Tarragon, Shallot, Sorrel, Chive, Nutmeg, and Horse Radish.** Natural honey is fine too. His favorite herb for menopause is **Sage** because "of its richness in female hormones". **Red Grape** leaves which accelerate the circulation through foot-baths; good for face flushes and hypertension also. Prepare the bath with a gallon of water in which you boil 2 - 3 handsful of leaves for 10 - 15 minutes. He lists also a recipe for a decoction to treat sudden flushes and high blood pressure:

Rosemary	-	*50 grains*
Mint	-	*30 grains*
Elecampane	-	*25 grains*
Mugwort	-	*25 grains*
St. John's Wort	-	*25 grains*
Shepherd's Purse	-	*25 grains*
Vervain	-	*25 grains*
Oak Apples	-	*25 grains*

grain : 480 grains/oz.

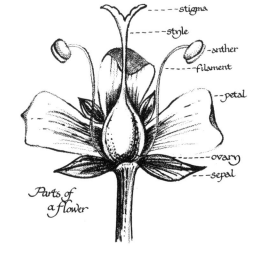

Parts of a flower

stigma

style

anther

filament

petal

ovary

sepal

He suggests you take a quart of boiling water. Let stand overnight with one handful of the mixture within. In the morning, strain it and take for 10 days in a row. Then rest for 2 days, and repeat.

A recipe given anonymously and handed out through our local Women's Center is:

Tea for Hormone Imbalance as Produced in Menopause -
One part each: **Sarsaparilla, Licorice, Blue Vervain.**
If serious add: one part each of **false unicorn root** or **raspberry leaves.**

Again, those of us who are pre-menopausal (how about that as a new way to consider oneself!), can help change our culture's obsession with youth and the valuing of women as sexual objects by appreciating our elders right here and now. Seek out those sisters of ours who are in the middle years and affirm their beauty. What is more ridiculous than the mini-skirted grandmother? We women who neglect to say how beautiful the aging process really is for women are paving the fall for ourselves as well. We're not in the habit of honoring our elders. Our very wise old women would not try to be young if we but appreciated them as they are. There are other purposes to life than bearing children and being the attractive appendages to men;[9] we all know this. Yet is is our menopausal sisters that are now fully experiencing this. Let us aid them in this self-discovery by sharing our respect, and love, for older women.

1. Osawa, Airola, Ehret, etc.
2. Or the reverse! Keen interest in sex, for some women, as this is the first time to explore one's sexuality without the fear of pregnancy.
3. Menopause is an **initiation** and we should not forego this just because men don't consider **their** menopause as important.
4. New England Journal of Medicine, Dec. 4, 1973, Lancet, April 14, 1973; Annals of Western Medicine and Surgery, Vol. 4, 1950, New York State Journal of Medicine, May 15, 1952.
5. Ursula Le Guin first used this term in conjunction with a menopausal woman in an article entitled, "The Space Crone".
5A. Some writers state that in a "healthy" woman, (e.g. Bieler, Kulvinkas), the ovaries never quit functioning; a woman will continue to be fertile long after her "unhealthy" sisters are finished with their menopause.
6. British Medical Journal, October 18, 1975.
7. Betty Lee Morales, July 1976, "Let's Live" magazine.
8. Herbal Remedies II, Family Press, Salt Lake City, Utah 1975.
9. Paavo Airola says about this: "Menopause is a divinely designed phase in woman's life, with a purpose of liberating her from duties as procreator with God, and giving her time for self-improvement, for the perfection of her human and divine characteristics, and her spiritual growth". From July 1976, "Let's Live" magazine in an excellent article entitled, "Menopause: Dreadful Affliction or Glorious Experience - Nutritional and Other Biological Solutions to Menopausal Problems, Estrogen Therapy, and Premature Aging".

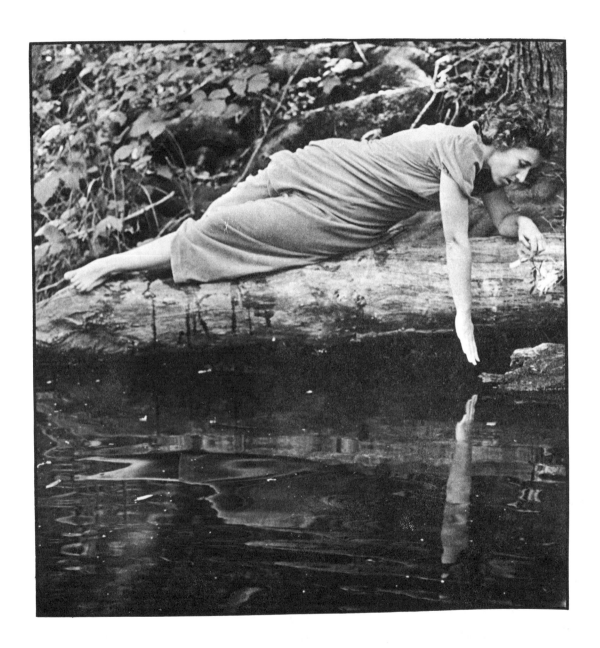

There were three goddesses in the Greek heavens who were never touched by Aphrodite, the goddess of love.

First was Hestia who was the first-born and last-born of her parents (for her father, old Chronos, swallowed her first after birthing and then disgorged his children, Hestia being the last). She was courted by Poseidon, Lord of the Oceans, and Apollo, twin to Artemis—and refused them downright to tend the sacred hearths, chaste all her life.

Second was Athena, born from Zeus's head in battle cry and full regalia. She cares nothing of men and spends her time in clever spinnings, always crafty and very wise. Third was Artemis, huntress enough to win the moon from Selene. She is the ecstatic dancing mother Bly speaks about. The one virginal, not in any means through lack of passion or cunning or chase, but in the sense that she never has a child. There are all manner of ways to be fertile. The obvious is undergoing a re-visioning of sorts. The ancients are being revalued. Rheia, the old Earth Mother cannot survive the softening of her sons. The birth of a child now is more than the gods' opinion that life should go on. The patterns reflected by stories the Greeks told give substance to our smelting of half-baked visions & alchemical intuitions. Being infertile, in our present day, is not so much unlike Hestia, Athena & Artemis. An ideology, i.e. feminism supports this way of being in the world. There are all manner of ways to be infertile as well. All ways, the choice is ours if we but accept the dream of being "doer." Infertility/fertility: like the cycle of being asleep & awakening. Who holds us in our infertility, our times of creative barreness, like Hades holds his sons, Sleep & Death, with him in the underworld? In the dark, Sleep touches the lives of us mortals. But once Death touches us, the dream is over. Infertility, such phases as I've experienced, awakens my fear of death. An ancient one, a present one. When I am touched by Aphrodite, the desire to confront Death is born. Imagined through to orgasm, completes but one spiral in Love's dance. For to come full circle, I must meet Persephone not here in the springtime of spirit but in the abode of the Soul, in the winter of femininity (the menopause). Let us remember to end our exploration of infertility with the menopause.

Though I do not know how the gods will receive you, the I Ching reminds you not to put on false appearances before God. When menopause means the cessation of fertility, we are freed from our desire to share a baby space with others. Now is the time of greatest pauses in our lives. This goes for men as well as women. The great and powerful binds of attachment and the years of being householders are coming to an end. Children are grown. Our paths change. The old gods are re-examined. Saturn makes the second return to his natal place. The night of the journey is beginning, and we start this time in complete honesty. No need to pretend fertility now. Persephone is underground this season. The dance of estrogen moves from a strutting to a self-reflection. Sitting still, the zinc will not settle nor the copper shine too highly, and with time, we will learn to balance between our living and our dying.

My first awareness of menopause was within my family. Watching our older aunts go through a change, and/or resist this natural process. At sixteen I was writing sentences in short stories like, "...the menopausal hens cackled." I saw this future experience as another aspect of female sexuality; anticipated with as much pleasure/pain as all the rest. I like Ursula Le Guin saying it's our opportunity to finally become crones. Sounds pedestrianly golden. Menopause, experienced fully (obviating the need for medicinal technological aids), seemed part and parcel of completing the owner's or operator's instructions when I took this female package out 28 years ago.

It is feeling more and more presumptuous on my part to be writing about menopause when I've just confessed my age. I'm barely a pubescent, in my evolutionary consciousness myself. Espousing to come from my own experience all previous notes are fantasies. Please regard the recipes and manufacturer's instructions on how to operate your self (body) according to current health, herbal and nutritional mythologies, as such.

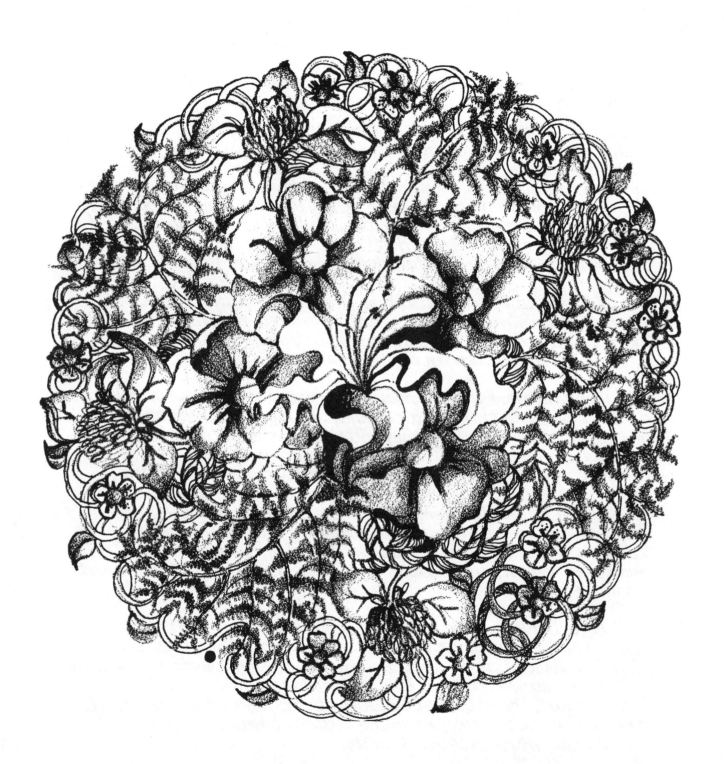

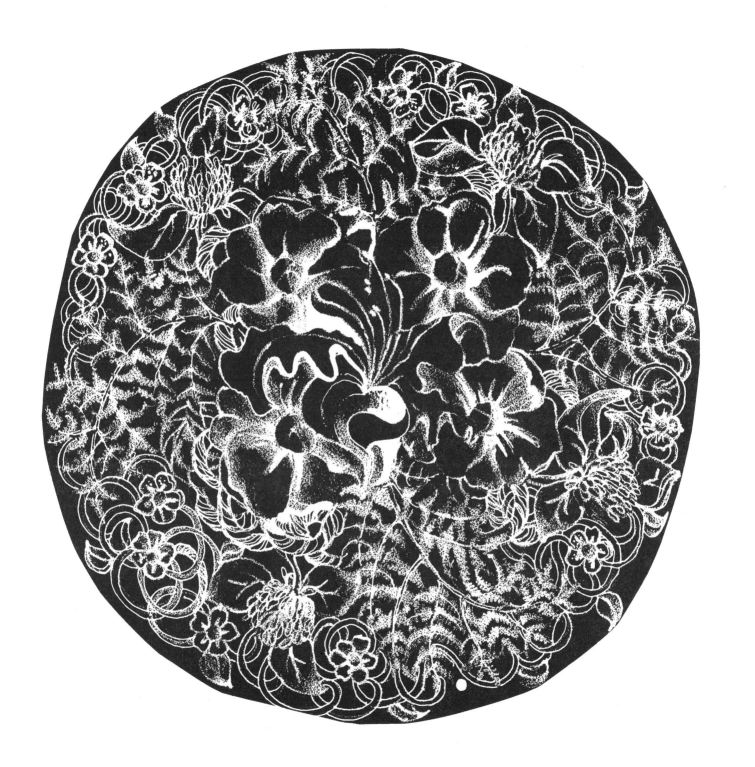

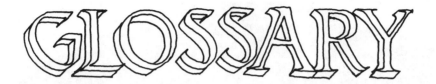

GLOSSARY

ABORTION - *The termination of pregnancy in the early stages. The death of the embryo.*

ACCEPTANCE – *Bufu said, "The final test isn't death, it's acceptance without proof."*

AFFIRMATIONS - *Prayer, self-suggestion for a positive goal. The repetition of what you desire. A mantra; energy follows thought.*

AFFLICTION - *In astrology, the difficult relationship between planets of 90 or 180°.*

ALCHEMY - *The meeting of magic and science whose creative child is named Truth.*

ALLOPATHIC *Rational medicine, as opposed to wholistic healing.*

ALLY - *Friend, one who guides.*

AMENORRHEA - *The absence of menstrual flow.*

AMNIOTIC - *The sea which contains the embryo; the first fluid, this "bag-of-waters".*

ANAPHRODISIAC - *A substance which dampens sexual desire.*

AQUARIAN - *Of the zodiac sign Aquarius, of the 11th house, ruled by Uranus. The "New-Age" - consciousness of sharing as sisters and brothers, ideals and hopes.*

ART - *The child of Eros and Psyche - of love and soul. The creative process. Passion contained.*

ASANA - *"Seat" - posture, pose. Placing the body/mind consciously in formal seating before God.*

ASTROLOGY - *The study of stars. As above, so below. A science of many faces - empirical, esoteric, medical, spiritual, humanistic, feminist, mundane, horary, and even the prenatal epoch, or conscious conception can be understood by this study.*

AVATAR - *A holy being who reincarnates to our Earth to inspire humans towards God.*

AWARENESS - *Consciousness, open attention, equated with Here/Now.*

A BABY - *The being who contains yourself; one very fresh from God. Newcomer to our planet.*

BAND-AIDS - *Topical treatment for hurts, soothing the obvious symptom.*

BASAL BODY TEMPERATURE - *The reflection of your internal fire via a slender glass cylinder holding Mercury.*

*The temperature graph reads but a personal fertility dance, feverish crescendo after the peak of ovulation!
Good to use when first beginning natural birth control in order to give empirical support for your intuitive knowledge
about fertility.*

BELLY - *Abdomen, the area within the pelvis. Tummy. Source of power below solar plexus - the womb. When
bellies are bleeding, a woman is so powerful that men fear her still.*

BIRTH - *Childbirth; the other side of death; coming in. Life's oldest ritual.*

BLEEDING - *Indians say, "in her moon"; menstruation; menses; menarche. Also, if excessive, called hemorrhage, wherein
much blood flows from the body. It is possible to hemorrhage from the vagina. Stop it immediately and uncover
the reason, e.g. retained placenta, blood poisoning, etc.*

BODY - *The most material illusion of all. What our awareness operates through and is always reflected on,
by environment; the temple of the soul.*

BRAIN - *In our heads, the location of the hypothalamus, pituitary and other vital governing glands and systems.
It is our heaviest organ, mind-stuff.*

BRAHMACHARYA - *Marriage to God; the application of Self-Control, or celibacy in householding, joining together
only to produce children.*

BREASTFEEDING - *Lactation , nursing, giving titty. The process of nourishing offspring which completes a
woman's fertility cycle when she's sexual.*

BREATH - *Prana; the wind of the goddesses. The stuff mind follows to the Heart.*

BREECH - *Feet first upon emergence from the Mother. Babaji says breech babies are healers.*

BREW *A tea; warmed drink or broth. Sometimes medicinal, always presented with graciousness and steeped
with love. Can be cold, too.*

BRIS - *The Jewish custom of slicing/tearing off the foreskin of a newborn's penis, usually at eight days of age.
Then he can go to heaven.*

BUMP - *An eruption on the skin, tiny metaphor for disruption of the inscape, may refer to warts, chancres, blisters,
pimples, pustules, boils, etc.*

CALMATIVE - *Any substance which has a quieting calming effect. Music and massage are good examples of this
as well as herbal brews.*

CANCER - *The epidemic disease of imperialistic countries; uncontrolled growth in humanistic tradition responding
well to meditation, visualization, diet, fasting, psychic healing, etc.*

CELEBRATION - *The spontaneous fulfillment of joy's potential. Opportunities are ever present at conceptions,
birthings, puberty, menopause, and dyings.*

CERVIX - *Literally, the "neck" in Latin; the lower and slightly elongated neck of the womb; has a psychosexual connection with the throat. What opens (the process of dilating) during the first stage of labor.*

CHAUVINIST - *One who is sexist; prejudiced person, especially towards women (or sometimes towards other nationalities; bigot).*

CHILDBIRTH - *Birth; the delivery from the heavens to the material. Baby space traveler arrives on the scene. A meeting of souls in passageways. Feels the same as death, vibrationally.*

CIRCLE - *The form of all things. One night, many moons ago, I dreamed of being embraced by a very wise, old woman. My guide. She whispers in my ear as we begin to twirl - "I will teach you the secret of circles!!!" Up and up we go til we soar . . GREY HAIRED ELDER, SPIN ME!*

CLITORIS - *The organ of pleasure in the female covered by a foreskin; above the vagina.*

COLIC - *Spasms, usually painful, in the intestines or belly. The manifestation of tensions reflecting the need for wiser nourishments. Feet rubs (reflexology) as well as soothing mealtimes work well with herbal treatments. Avoid drastic changes in temperature.*

COLVILLE INDIANS - *From Washington State, their reservation had built upon it the Grand Coulee Dam. Now they want their land back. My father says our people never declared war on the United States, but now it is time to reclaim our heritage, and our Land.*

CONCEPTION - *"Conception is an act of God and needs no proof". Baba Hari Das writes in a personal letter. This word has changed meaning in the 20th century with the advent of mass technological birth control. Whereas it used to mean the meeting of sperm and egg, or fertilization, it now means the implantation in the uterus of the zygote, or fertilized egg. In this way, the Pill and the I.U.D. can still be classified as "contraceptives" rather than abortifacients.*

CONSCIOUS CONCEPTION - *The term I'd like to see replace "natural birth control". The calling in of the life force with respect, resulting in pregnancy. Implies a non-violent approach to family planning.*

CONSCIOUSNESS - *The projection of time upon the aggregate of senses, the body; upon the environment, which is earth, air, water and fire (including other people); and upon the mind, which is a process of correlating information. Awareness; transmits via the senses "facts" or relative truths.*

CONTAINER - *A vessel; that which holds and gives form by its own material shape. Containers in our bodies are lungs (breath), skull (brains), and womb (babies or blood).*

CONTRACEPTION - *Against conception; though in our culture, refers to an agent which kills .*

CONTRACTIONS - *In reference to the uterus, powerfully coordinated muscle movements of the womb; a rush of energy through the uterus; the opposite to release and/or expansion.*

CRAMPS - *Actually uterine contractions which contain a build-up of lactic acid (and possibly other toxic substances - by products of cell metabolism or pollution). Cramps call attention to the need for relaxation with conscious breathing and a gentle movement or change in position.*

CUNT - *Vagina; puss(y), "down-there", nooky, birth opening. Where blood flows out during menstruation and penises come in during coitus. A "swear", "dirty", "cuss" and/or "bad" word currently being re-imagined by feminists.*

CYCLE - *As in "menstrual cycle", "fertility cycle" and "bi-o-cycle". The experience of wholeness, knowledge of the circle; mandala consciousness. As opposed to linear reality, rationalism - like, just ask a medical technician when the menstrual cycle begins - there's no answer.*

CYST - *A collection of fluid around an organ e.g. ovarian cyst. The metaphoric statement concerns containment, holding back, and/or security-protection.*

DECOCTION - *A process of taking out of herbs their medicinal properties.*

DELIVERY - *Meeting a baby in the human dimension of consciousness. Generally referred to as the emergence of a baby from the birth opening.*

DE-TOXIFICATION - *Purification; the process of cleansing; removal of poisons.*

DOUCHE - *The cleansing of the vagina inside by way of a flow of liquid, with or without medicinal value. A container (douche bag - bladder of some animal, etc.), a nozzle and a valve are helpful in transporting the fluid into the vagina.*

ECOBOLIC - *A drug that accelerates delivery by uterine contractions during birthing.*

EDIFICATION - *A fancy word for enjoyment that may be educational too.*

EGG - *The ovum; a woman's seed. The origin, the source, that which contains life-force. (See Meditations on Conception in the appendix.)*

EMMENAGOGUE - *A substance which induces menstrual flow; like herbs, prayer, etc.*

EMPIRICISM - *True science based on experience. Does not deny the subjective in its theory. All witches were empiricists as opposed to their tormentors, who were rationalists.*

EROS - *The force of love; in Greek mythology, the son of Aphrodite and Ares (the Goddess of Beauty and the God of War). He was exquisite and attended by Pothos (Longing) and Himeros (Desire): worshipped by all of us when in love.*

ESTROGEN - *A hormone, or chemical message secreted by the ovaries in a female. Men have this female hormone to a lesser degree, unless he practices yoga, drinks licorice tea, and/or smokes dope.*

FASTING - *Resting the digestive system and giving a chance to the eliminative systems to really clean oneself.*

Recommended at the beginning of menstruation, during labor and directly after birthing. Not recommended while pregnant or breastfeeding (for prolonged periods of time).

FECUNDITY *- Fertile, fertility. Able to reproduce, become pregnant, full of potential, richness, luxuriousness.*

FEELINGS *- Associated with our brain-heart as opposed to emotions which are a function of the mind. What brings our senses to the Here/Now. Very fluctuating in pregnancy and just before menstruation and high during ovulation in women.*

FEMALE *- The aspect of universal energy which creates; feminine; women and girls.*

FEMINIST *- A woman/girl/person who defines themselves by their own experience. A woman identified woman. One who chooses to fully participate in living.*

FERTILE *- Fertility - Able to create, to be with child, fecund. In women (and also men), this is a cyclical function. When other animals (mammals) are in their periods of fertility, they are called "in heat" - woman's temperature raises when fertile, too during ovulation phase.*

FERTILIZATION *- The union of the male element (energy) with the female (creativity) resulting in something new - a baby (zygote), an idea, an art form.*

FETUS *- The baby growing within after the embryonic stage. A sentient being. Each fetus is the Christ-child (or any avatar of your choosing). Handle with care.*

FOCUS *- Concentrating energy; looking clearly and precisely; powerful attention.*

FURIES *- Roman goddesses of vengeance who live in Erebus, the darkness below Hades through which all the dead must pass.*

FOMENTATION *- An application of moisture with heat to reduce swelling and ease pain.*

FUCKING *- The process of joining together the female and male reproductive organs; coitus; sexual intercourse; another "naughty" word needing to be re-imagined. The power is given by mystifying and punishing this natural physical expression. We can re-claim the power for positive means by being responsible in our own fucking relationships without embarrassment.*

GALACTAGOGUE *- An agent which stimulates or increases the flow of milk.*

GEOCENTRIC *- Regarding the universe as centered about one's self on Earth. The natal horoscope of an individual is geocentric, for example.*

GERM THEORY *- An idea that microscopic (invisible to our unaided eyes) entities cause illness and can be transmitted from one person to another, called contagion.*

GESTATION *- The time of formation within; pregnancy; being with child; knocked up.*

GIRL - *A female child; female before maturity, which can come during puberty rites of passage. In this culture,, the feeling of being a woman is attached in relationship with men. I.E., the celebration of marriage rituals. This is unfortunate. Initiation into womanhood could come during menstruation or via our elder women. A girl may change into a woman through the experience of childbirth. But this isn't always the case either. Try to pinpoint in your own life emergence as a woman from being a little girl.*

GRAIN-OF-SALT - *Always use sparingly; the information qualified in such a way means "use carefully". Be your own empiricist and feel from the inside if it's true.*

GRIPING - *Painful contractions of the intestines, similar to colic. Sometimes it's the breaking down of hard adhesions to intestinal walls. Fomentations help, as do breathing in relaxation and no resistance to the process.*

GROUNDED - *Of the Earth; open channel of cosmic energy yet of the Earth; feet on the ground, in touch with the material and aware of the spiritual.*

GYNECOLOGIST - *One who is knowledgable of pathological conditions in the female organs and is learning* **process** *from those of us who support this profession.*

GYNECOLOGY - *The study of the female reproductive/sexual systems. Any of us who take Socrates' maxim to "know thyself" will become gynecologists of Self.*

HADES - *King of the Underworld; swallowed at birth by his father, Chronos, and rescued by Zeus; Pluto, whose kingdom contained all lost souls and the gods of Sleep and Death. He abducted Persephone and fed her the pomegranate, forever bonding her to cyclically return to the underworld (in the "dead of winter").*

HEALTH - *Not a state but a dynamic process of living in harmony with nature and balancing the elements of earth, water, air and fire within and without.*

HEART - *The destination of my Fall. Associated in the physical body with pumping of blood; in the subtle body as the seat of the soul (thymus). A baby's thymus gland is enormous - and a baby's mind is quieter (less chill). We know that breath brings mind to the Heart - the result is bliss.*

HEAVEN - *The environment of a mind happy and peaceful. Associated with the air element, being high, and in opposition to hell. The white light.*

HELL - *The abode of Hades; the Underworld; the deepest dark within. This is the place souls go, abandoning all hope. Sleep and Death live there too.*

HERB - *A weed that has been recognized as beneficial to humankind. A special plant which enriches our lives by the relationship.*

HERBOLOGY - *The study of plants and their uses. Classification according to families, results, and ancestral information is part of this science.*

HERSTORY - *Originally a pun on "history" showing the way our past has been recorded, herstory now describes* *any story told by a female; the feminine of history.*

HORMONE - *From the Greek word meaning to stimulate, any substance produced by a gland (an organ that secretes) which has a specific effect when carried via the bloodstream to another organ. The same definition for plants.*

HOUSEHOLDER - *One who inhabits a house on the Earth while living with God in her heart, or the Goddess in her soul. A difficult sadhana (spiritual practice). In India, one on a spiritual path would be a householder for the first part of the adult life and then become devoted to a solitary practice during the latter years. Sometimes the world catches us though.*

HYGIEIA - *The Greek Goddess of Health. I chose a Greek because those of us living in the western world still enact the Greek myths daily.*

HYPOTHALAMUS - *The gland below the thalamus in the brain which is integral to any understanding of the female reproductive cycle, feelings, and higher consciousness.*

HYSTERIA - *From the Greek word meaning "suffering in the womb" but taken to mean by psychiatry as any outbreak of wild, uncontrollable excitement or the unconscious simulation of organic disorders.*

IATROGENIC - *My Webster's New World Dictionary adds to the usual definition:* **especially of imagined symptoms;** *caused by the physician himself.*

IMAGINATION - *The process of seeing in the mind; from imago, the Latin for image and an imago is an adult insect in its reproductive stage of development; the power of creating something new by visualizing mentally something that is not here in the material world.*

IMPREGNANTE - *To make pregnant; to fertilize; to fill with ideas or feelings as well as with developing offspring.*

INFANTICIDE - *The murder of a baby.*

INFUSION - *The liquid extract which results from steeping a substance in water.*

INITIATION - *The ceremony by which one is introduced into a new phase of study and/or development.*

INTUITION - *The direct knowing without conscious reasoning; a process which relies on experience and perceptions rather than theories or concepts. A force women are given to understand.*

INVOLUTION - *The process of the uterus returning to its pre-pregnant size after the delivery of the placenta (or third stage of labor). Called after-contractions.*

IRREGULAR - *Not conforming to the established rule.*

ISOLATION - *To set apart from others; a process of being alone. Important during menses.*

ISHTAR - *A Babylonian Goddess of Fertility, special to the Moon and the Herbs.*

IX U SIHNAL - *Mayan Moon Goddess who ruled the birthing process.*

JANUS - *The Greek God who watches over comings and goings; guardian of passageways; two faced one. Reminding us that when the birth door opens, so does the exit towards death. On Earth we can balance between the two.*

JUNO - *A goddess of marriage. Queen of all the goddesses, married to Jupiter; very jealous. Associated with the Greek goddess, Hera. It is said that the Milky Way in the heavens are the droplets of milk spraying out from Juno's breasts.*

KAMASUTRA - *A Hindu manual on the art of love written in the eighth century.*

KAREZZA - *Literally caress, in Italian. Westernized Tantra. Friction and weaving of souls during the sexual embrace without orgasms. Non-seminal intercourse.*

KALI - *The aspect of Durga, the Divine Mother, in the form that destroys life as well as gives life. The age we are now in: Kali Yuga.*

KARMA - *From the Sanskrit meaning a deed, or fate. In Buddhism and Hinduism, the concept of reaping what one sows; cosmic cause and effect, influencing one through many lifetimes.*

KIRILIAN PHOTOGRAPHY - *Allowing us to see in pictures the colors of the auras which are energy fields surrounding all animate things. The life-force field as captured on celluloid by a process Kirilian discovered this century.*

LABOR - *The process of working to deliver a baby, toiling while opening up. Usually means the first part of childbirth, first and second stages. To develop in too great detail, i.e. to labor a point.*

LACTATION - *The period of time in which the young are nourished by the mother through secretion of milk in the mammary gland. Even dolphins lactate, her young having the milk propelled into their mouths by powerful, projectile breasts.*

LAMINARIA - *A seaweed that comes pre-packaged in hard slender sticks used for dilation of the cervical (opening) before abortions (D & C's, dilation and cutterage)*

LANGUAGE - *A special set of symbols (words, gestures, sounds) used for transmitting information. Shapes our world - view and cognitive processes. The power of language is obvious during altered states of consciousness like at birthings. My obstetrician friend said one "lady" he helped birth, complained during the crowning of her babies head that she was too small and needed an episiotomy. He watched her then tear exactly in the place where an episiotomy would be cut on her perineum! Watch out for what you order via the power of the spoken word. You can actually create accidents for your children by saying, "Be careful. You'll hurt yourself! Watch out, etc."*

LATIN - *A dead language which we resurrect through mythology and religion, the language of the ancient Romans. Also, one who lives in Latin America, or south of the United States on the American continent.*

LETTING GO - *Allowing, no attachment, surrendering to the flow (the Tao, God's plan, etc.). Exhalation, little dyings and death.*

LEUCOCYTE - A white blood cell which is in our tissues, blood and lymph. These colorless corpuscles are important in the body's defenses against infection (contamination with disease). Leucocytes also eat sperm. Leucocytes are also considered toxins due to an overabundance of undigested proteins.

LEUKORRHEA - "The Whites", profuse discharge from the vagina.

LIMBIC SYSTEM - A more "primitive" section of the brain in which "thinking" is not important. See the appendix on the Hypothalamus and other hormones.

LITURGICAL CHANTS - Repetition songs to awaken the Divine in man - in Latin, yet any song of the heart, be it Hindu or American Indian, can bring isolated individuals into a union with their fellow worshipers and with God.

LUMINARY - Here meant as the Moon and the Sun, but any body which gives light, like your yoga teacher.

LUMINOUS - Shining.

MAMMARY - The metaphor of nourishment in the female bodies of mammals, a classification of animals based on titty.

MANDALA - Exteriorization of the wholeness of consciousness; the circular form filled and emptied for meditation. The birth opening at crowning is a mandala for midwives, the cervix, as seen with speculum and flashlight is a mandala for all women.

MASECTOMY - The removal via surgery of the mammary tissue in women. Avoid at all possible costs! When Jaqueline Kennedy was having cesareans, it was the chic way to experience childbirth. Now with the new political wives undergoing radical masectomies (complete removal of the entire mammary gland), this operation is again gaining public favor as a means to rid oneself of cancer of the breasts. (See glossary for "cancer" definitions)

MAYAN - An ancient culture of Middle America (Latin) whose matriarchal nature is just being re-discovered through honoring their goddesses.

MEDICAL - MEDICINAL - Any process or substance used for treating disease. Appropriate to the realm of pathology, the study of suffering. Generally a science. It can be an art of healing. But the medicine woman has to be harmless herself, and do no harm.

MEDITATION - Many forms of this knowing oneself. Mothers may meditate on diaper changing as their spiritual practice; i.e. full attention on just what you are doing. The outcome is an elevation of a mundane task into a divine service, and no soft babies ever stuck by pins.

MENARCHE - MENSES - MENSTRUATION - Three words to describe a woman in her moon; the shedding of the endometrium of the uterus which occurs when fertile yet not pregnant; "on the rag"; having a period; being visited by "my little friend"; purification; renewal.

MATRIX - Greek for womb.

MENOPAUSE - *The time of cessation of menstruations; the pause in fertility; the last aspect of sexuality (puberty/ menstruation the 1st, menses/pregnancy the 2nd, childbirth and nursing the 3rd). When in good health, a blessing.*

POINT - MIDPOINT - *A calculation on the natal horoscope (generally) to indicate what constitutes predispositions of weaknesses, confluences and symbols or relationship between planets and other life-support systems.*

MIDWIFE - *Facilitates the birthing, usually of a baby, by her patient presence. Support and knowledge gently balanced. We are all giving birth our selves each moment.*

MINDFULNESS - *Fully present; having in mind totally; awareness in depth; a style of meditation.*

MIND'S EYE - *The imagination.*

MINERALS - *Any substance, organic or inorganic, of the earth; bodies contain minerals, yet are classified as animals rather than vegetable or mineral.*

MISCARRIAGE - *The cessation of pregnancy; carrying a baby ends with a stillbirth. Generally applied in definition to the middle or later time of gestation. "Nature's way of correcting a mistake."*

the MOTHER - *Of many forms, like meditation. She can be the Good Mother (Dancing, Ecstatic, Virginal) or the Bad Mother (the Death Mother, the Dark). A woman who has born a child; that which is the origin, with authority and responsibility for this relationship; a term used as a title of respect; affectionately, and sometimes for the elders amongst us, and the ones before.*

MOTHERLOVE - *A feeling of unconditional loving; a desire to nurture and protect one's young. Not limited to women bearing children, by any means. I invite you to practice with my young, all our children.*

MYSTERY - *Anything that remains unknown or secret which excites curiosity. As Uranus transits Scorpio, no wonder this book came to be?!*

MYSTIFY - *To involve with mystery, to deliberately bewilder; to perplex or puzzle; leaving loose ends behind (a great help in childbirth).*

MYTH - *Any imaginary person or thing; a traditional story or collection of tales told to explain the natural mysteries of birth, and creation, and death, and love, etc.*

MYTHOLOGY - *The study of myth-making and our own parts in the play. My mythos, is author - your's is reader. For this generation, the Edipus/Electra myth doesn't fit anymore - what is the present one now unfolding?*

NADIR - *The lowest point on the mandala of consciousness. Due south, towards the depths of soul. In astrology, the cusp of the fourth house, wherein the crab, motherly attachments, naturally live.*

NAPKIN - *Here used to describe a sanitary pad or a diaper. Something material which collects and contains eliminations from the pelvic floor. My current favorite sanitary napkin is a piece of cotton batting (I once collected cotton off the plants in central California, removed the seeds and other hard materials from it that very winter, and used it to stuff our herbal pillows.) I cover the cotton with any beautiful scrap of material, saved from old clothes primarily. Then, when filled with blood, I bury, or burn the napkin. Return it to the mother. Napkins wipe lips, just like our mamas did for us.*

NATAL - *Of birth; concerned with the moment of individuality; in astrology, the basic map of one's soul evolution. A natal chart is a horoscope.*

NATURAL - *Of or arising from nature; real, as found in nature. Baba Hari Das has commented that yoga isn't natural for men whereas sex is.*

NATURAL BIRTH CONTROL - *Sexual beings reporting their experiences of fertility via a methodology; using no mechanical or chemical tools from technological medicine to avoid conceptions. Presently, the methods known to this author are: lunaception, basal body temperature, mucus (Billings or "ovulation method"), dreams, tarot, I Ching, and astrology (and other sciences of the occult), herbs, nutrition, body work (polarity, Reichian, bio-energetics and other tools for increasing awareness of one's sexual flow), Karezza, Tantra Yoga, Psychic, and total mothering via breastfeeding, sleeping, etc. with existing offspring. Like to see this term re-defined as "conscious conception".*

NECTAR - *From the Greek, that which overcomes death; a drink of the Gods & Goddesses; also the sweet fluid found in flowers and made into honey by bees; any tea you may brew when you also put in your love.*

NEW AGE - *The age of Aquarius wherein we have heaven here on earth; wherein we realize our hopes and ideals; wherein we view people as divine beings, as brothers and sisters, and not as objects for manipulation, sexually or otherwise. The time/space projected by consciousness of equality and androgyny.*

NIGGER - *Black person; white person jiving black, black person passing for white; an archaic derogatory term for one of African descent and dark pigmentation.*

NUCLEAR FAMILY - *Mother, father and children living in isolation; schizogenetic situation labeled "normal" and "the American way". Breeding ground for ignorance, angst (existential anxiety) and possessiveness.*

NURSING - *From the Latin, to nourish; to feed at the breast; the act of suckling.*

OBSTETRICS - *The area of medicine that concerns itself with diagnosing and treating diseases of pregnancy, childbirth and the immediate post-partum time. We pay our obstetricians to be paranoid for us. However when the natural process isn't interested with, or breaks down, their services are not needed. Some obstetricians are midwives. I've met two in seven years of going to birthings.*

OVULATION - *The process of releasing a mature female germ cell from the ovary. Refers to the entire time of fertility immediate to the bursting through of the graafian follicle by the ovum.*

OXYTOCIC - *Having an effect produced by oxytocin.*

OXYTOCIN - *A hormone released by the pituitary gland and affecting the smooth muscle tissue in the uterus;*

causes contractions and/or expulsive movements of the womb; ecobolic. Produced via stimulation to the breasts by nursing or by an infant sniffing the undersides of nipples.

PARTHENOGENESIS - Literally, *virgin origin*. Reproduction by an unfertilized yet developing ovum. Androgyny conceives itself. The women being pregnant without a man's sperm, totally of Herself.

PARTUITION - The process of giving birth; delivery.

PATRIARCHY - From the Greek meaning "father-rule"; a form of social organization in which the father is the head and the rules dominated by men; consider the current health care and their supporting institutions.

PERINEUM - "T'aint the puss and t'aint the asshole". *Southern folk saying.* The small area between the vagina and the anus; the womb of the shakti wherein Kundalini lies sleeping; muladhara chakra. Daily massage and/or yogic practice in this area reduces tearing or need for episiotomy during crowning and delivery of a baby.

PERCEPTION - A function of the brain-heart; to grasp or take in mentally; an insight to become aware through the senses and reflect on the relative truths.

PERIOD - A Greek word meaning "around-way" period, a cycle; appearing at regular intervals; occurring from time to time; a portion of time distinguished by certain processes; the menses; an end or conclusion.

PHILOSOPHY - The study of the underlying systems of thought which give knowledge of the universe; from the Greek meaning wise-loving.

PITUITARY - The master sex gland producing many hormones vital for reproduction. Right next to the hypothalamus, the seat of emotions. The link between feelings and sexuality.

PLACENTA - The afterbirth; the organ which respires and cleanses the baby's bloodstream; delivered in the final stage of birthing. (See placenta recipes.)

POLLUTION - To make impure, corrupt, unclean; by-product of greed and non-loving lifestyles.

POULTICE - An application of a softened pulp or mass, usually warmed and layered on a soreness of the body.

PRANA - The vital life-force which is charged with divine energy by the sun; each inhalation brings prana inside our beings to re-vitalize us.

PRANAYAMA - The science and practice of conscious breath control.

PREGNANCY - To be with child growing within one's uterus; to be mentally fertile and yielding of creative thought; to be fruitful; full of meaning.

PREJUDICE - Preconceived idea, sometimes held despite the reality; harm resulting as from some action or judgment of another; hatred for other races.

PRIMITIVE - Primary; existing from the earliest ages; simple; original; pre-literate.

PROGESTERONE - *The hormone produced in greatest quantities in the pregnant woman; first released by the corpus luteum in the ovary and then by the placenta.*

PROHIBITION - *Literally before having: to refuse to permit; prevent; hinder.*

PROGRESSION - *In astrology, the moving forward of natal planets giving the individual accurate "birth-charts" for each moment of her life.*

PROLACTIN - *A hormone in breastfeeding women; the mothering hormone; given to roosters, they stop crowing and go sit on eggs.*

PROPAGATE - *To cause a plant or animal to reproduce herself. To extend or transmit through air or water.*

PSYCHE - *Soul; In Greek and Roman mythology, the one so beautiful that she was made immortal by Zeus. She is the mother of Delight (Voluptas) and wife of Eros. Her link with the soul is known not only with Greek and Roman mythology. James Hillman is doing much good work in bringing her back to psychology.*

PSYCHEDELIC - *Literally, to make manifest the soul; an agent which alters consciousness.*

PSYCHOLOGY - *The study of the human mind and behavior; a science of the subject.*

PSYCHOSEXUAL - *Having to do with the psychological aspects of sexuality much as body fantasy, etc.*

PUBERTY - *A rite of passage into reproductivity; in females, the onset of menses.*

PUBESCENT - *Having attained puberty; covered with soft down, plant or animal.*

PURGE - *To clean out; catharsis; to move through the being unwanted material; to rid oneself of guilt; to cause a thorough bowel movement.*

PURE - *Free from any contaminant; unadulterated, chaste; abstract; absolute.*

PUSS, PUSSY - *Slang for cunt.*

RADIATIONS - *The process of sending out rays of light, heat, energy; to give forth from a center. X-radiations are to be avoided, especially in the childbearing years and before. Always shield the ovaries when receiving x-rays!*

RATIONALISM - *The process of accepting Reason as the only correct choice for all decisions, beliefs, or behavior. As opposed to empiricism, which looks at the results of science, or the real world and listens to intuition and whatever else works or makes sense. Allopathy is a good example of rationalism.*

RELATIONSHIP - *The process by which the universe composes itself of equal beings. Kinship; being connected by blood or marriage or HEART.*

REPRODUCTION - *To bring forth more of its own kind, especially by sexual intercourse; the process of seeing beings who contain oneself - baby making.*

RHIZOME - *A creeping stem lying underneath the surface. It produces roots from the underside and sends aerial shoots above.*

RHYTHM - *Literally from the Greek, to measure the flow; a movement having a regularly repeated pattern of beats, accents; specific biological changes; in biology of periodic occurrances in living organisms.*

RITUAL - *Any formal, customary observance or practice of rites; ceremonial action with deeper meaning for participants. All of us, even the identified anarchists, practice rituals daily, most are unconscious however and have been set up for us through our ancestors and culture.*

ROOT - *The part of a plant which draws up (usually) nourishment from the soil; that part which does not have nodes, shoots or leaves and usually lies below the ground surface; an ancestor; the intimate connection one has with her place of birth, the people involved in one's upbringing, or any feelings of allegience through long association.*

SADHANA - *Spiritual practice in the Yogi tradition; for householders, one's sadhana is caring for children and creating and maintaining a beautiful and inspiring environment, called "house" or nest.*

SAMSKARA - *The impression upon the immortal soul of an individual which attracts certain experiences or people to her in the present. Samskara can be laid down during pregnancy, or through previous lifetimes.*

SCIENCE - *Originally, from the Latin, To Know; systemized knowledge derived from theory, observation, experimentation, and repeatability. The two main schools are empiricism and rationalism.*

SENSATION - *The process of receiving direct information through bodily stimulation. There are five acknowledged vehicles for this: eyes (sight), ears (hearing), skin (touch), tongue (taste) and nose (smell). Sensations of the mind may be called intuition.*

SENSUOUS - *Enjoying or easily stimulated by the senses, as distinguished from the intellect or spirit. Senses shroud the spirit in illusion.*

SEX - *The division of the One into two - male and female; with sex, comes death.*

SEXIST - *One who descriminates and oppresses persons of the opposite gender, usually men exploiting and socially domineering women.*

SILENCE - *Absence of any sound or noise; containment of vital energy. Every pregnant person should enjoy this state before their baby is born as much as possible because afterwards, silence becomes very precious.*

SMIDGEON - *Just a little bit; teensy weensy; small amount.*

SOUL - *Psyche; the part of one's being that is linked with the center of feeling, will, etc.; spiritual and emotional force; the part that lives on after death and reincarnates or chooses another body to return to the Earth. The shadow of the Spirit.*

SOUL-MAKING - *The process of exploring, deepening, and surrendering to one's dharma, or path as it is meant to be; what we do each time we fall in love.*

SPECULUM - *In medical technology, an instrument to dilate (open circularly) a passageway; the metal or plastic tool used to open up the vagina and see the cervix by means of a flashlight and mirror.*

SPERM , SPERMATAZOA - *The male germ cell; analagous to the egg in a man or fertile boy; contained in semen, the fluid which emits from the penis in ejaculation, usually at orgasm. It can penetrate the female germ cell creating another, a zygote. They are conscious beings!*

SPIRIT - *Latin for breath; synonymous with God, the Origin; the part that never dies or changes; the perfected Self; the essential nature of all things.*

STILLBORN - *A baby delivered dead; the soul chooses to leave the body at birth. Important to allow the mother to see and hold her stillborn, and say "good-by".*

STIMULATE - *From the Latin, to prick; to arouse, make excited; stir up or spur on; in medicine, to excite (an organ) to increase activity.*

STRESS - *A mental or physical strain; a force exerted on a body that deforms it; urgency, pressure; the cause of a great many illnesses. The antidote is yoga - changing our internal world to a more peaceful one, which will then reflect in an external world of less stress.*

STUDY - *The application of the mental processes to acquire knowledge and understand; when study affects the Heart, it is called wisdom.*

SUBTLE BODY - *Originally meaning, closely woven; "under a web"; when we pressed Babaji one day for a definition of this most tenuous concept, he replied, "The subtle body is the physical body without the physical body". This is our least gross aspect of our physical-emotional body and the part that is stimulated via pranyama and yoga asana. It is what astral travels during flying dreams in the nighttime.*

TAMPON - *When I was a teenager, this was synonymous with sanitary protection during menses. It is an internal plug that soaks up all your fluids and hides the fact that one is indeed menstruating. We lose power by pretending.*

TANTRIC - *One form of yoga which is very dangerous without proper instruction because it is very easy to get trapped by sex; try Karezza first.*

TEA - *An infusion of herbs and water by boiling the water, then pouring it over the herb (one teaspoon to a cup of water, app.). Steep in a covered container which is non-metallic (especially aluminum!). Then strain and serve as a beverage, or use the power of the sun or moon to make tea.*

TESTOSTERONE - TESTERONE - *The male sex hormone that is present in women when they do a regular yoga practice in a more balanced (sattvic) way. Like estrogen in its stimulation of aggression, but much more so. Grandfathers can nurse babies when their testosterone level decreases with aging: a crystaline steroid.*

TIT - *A slang term for breast and nipple and/or the giving of milk/nurturance from the breast; bosom; easiest of all words for a baby to pronounce.*

TONIC - *An agent that stimulates tissue nutrition and/or improves, invigorates, and/or restores the system. Especially good in the springtime, during that annual spring cleaning time.*

TOXEMIA - *A condition where poisonous substances are in the bloodstream; in pregnancy, a disease which gives danger signals of spots before the eyes, black-outs, rapid,weight gain, swelling of the ankles, etc. May be prevented by nutrition and other health considerations before and during gestation.*

TOXIN - *Any poison produced by plant, animal or micro-organism. Especially man in the 20th century.*

TRANSIT - *The apparent passage of a heavenly body over a certain meridian in astrology, the change of position of luminaries and planets which affect the natal chart of an individual. The study brings a sense of cyclical rhythm and meaning, plus transcendence, to one's life.*

TRUTH - *The quality of being in agreement with Reality; occurs at the meeting of space and time in experience of the relationship and "utter inter-dependence" of environment, mind and body.*

UMBILICAL CORD - *The life-line between a developing fetus and the placenta, or organ which nourishes and cleanses the baby. Out after birth, the baby is given the breast, as the external life-line - titty now acting as the placenta for the baby for the next nine months (at least) (hopefully).*

UNDERSTAND - *To know clearly and fully the nature of something; to support (standing under) the knowing with meaning.*

URANUS - *In Greek mythology, the God who was the Heavens and fathered the Titans, Furies, and Cyclops. The most ancient of the Gods. He was overthrown by Saturn (Chronos - Father Time). The seventh planet of the solar system associated with quick, electrifying changes and the New-Age.*

UTERUS - *Womb; our grounding; the hollow and muscularly powerful organ wherein the zygote attaches and grows till birthing; the monthly (or so) shedding of it's lining (endometrium) is called menstruation. THE CENTER.*

VAGINA - *In Latin, a sheath (for the sword that's called a penis?); the middle opening in the female's pelvic floor described from the vulva to the uterus; the canal is also called the vaginal barrel, which elongates during sexual excitement; a psycho-sexual link exists between the vagina and the mouth of an organism. The female sex organ; the birth canal. Called Yoni in Hindu mythology and revered as a symbol of the Creative.*

VEGETARIAN -*One who respects life-force and ahimsa, the path of non-violence. And/or one who only eats vegetables, grains, and seeds, nuts (perhaps fruit, too) for reasons of health. My rule is to eat things that don't have eyes (except potatoes!).*

VENUS - *The Roman Goddess of love and beauty (Greek: Aphrodite); Mother of Amor by Mars (Ares); Her festival dates are April 1 and August 19; the second planet in distance from the sun, whose transits always bring gifts from the goddesses.*

VESSEL - *A tube or duct circulating a bodily fluid; a container implying an opening; women are vessels for creativity, of which a baby is the grossest (most obvious and dense, or material) form.*

VIRGIN - *A maiden; a person, especially a female, who has not had sexual intercourse; unused, untrod, chaste. There are virgins however who do enjoy sex yet are pure unto themselves and form no attachments to their lovers - rare ones though.*

VIRGIN MARY - *The Mother of the Christ child; the Madonna (and every pregnant woman deserves this respect); the one who conceived without a man; the pure mother, whose son is martyred for the good of all God's children and the first Jewish mother!*

VISION - *The power of seeing; something seen by other than normal sight, e.g. in a dream, after a long fast, by force of imagination, in a trance-like quest for a personal image to guide one's life.*

VOMIT - *Matter thrown up from the stomach and out the mouth; babies do this easily and are great teachers in ridding one's body of* **undigested food** *due to its poor quality or feelings that came up and disrupted the digestive process.*

the WHITES - *Leukorrhea; vaginal discharge usually profuse (not the physiological message our body cyclically gives us about fertility).*

WITCH - *Originally from wicce, wise woman in her craft; a woman healer, usually an herbalist, and/or a midwife. Forerunners of our feminists - "Witch is to woman as womb is to birth". - Z. Budapest.*

WOMAN - *The female in the human species of animals; the girl growing up into a Goddess.*

WOMB - *The uterus; every person's first home (unless the vision of test-tube babies manifests); a woman's word for her source of power within her center.*

X-RAYS - *Radiations which affect developing germ cells in a negative way - can cause birth defects, even the "mild" ones used by medical and dentist's assistants. Always wear a shield of lead protecting the uterus and ovaries and surround yourself with impenetrable white and protecting light. Eating kelp is reported to help the thyroid deal with this invasion.*

YOGA - Union; the Yoke; a scientific and mystical practice towards self-realization and liberation (were every revolutionary a yogini first!). In the West, this practice has been popularized into gymnastics - however, yoga postures are but one of eight limbs to a complete and full understanding of God-nature within.

YOGINI - A female who practices yoga; more common now in the West as in India, women are discouraged from practicing yoga by their husbands. A good Hindi wife serves her husband as lord and master - a good yogini is married to God.

YONI - The Sanskrit word for vagina; symbol is an inverted triangle and is used in deep meditations called yantra.

ZENITH - The heights; in astrology, the midheaven or top of the chart; the cusp of the tenth house; directly opposite to the nadir.

ZYGOTE - The fertilized ovum; the creation of a third from two, the egg and the sperm; after fertilization occurs in the fallopian tube, the zygote travels to the receptive lining in the womb and attaches, wherein it is re-defined as an embryo. The beginning.

BIBLIOGRAPHY

Abel, E.L., *Moon Madness*. A Fawcett Gold Medal Book, 1977.

Airola, Paavo, *How to Get Well*. Health Plus Publishers, P.O. Box 22001, Phoenix, Arizona 85028, 1974.

. *Sex and Nutrition*. Phoenix: Health Plus Publishers, 1974.

. *Are You Confused?* Phoenix: Health Plus Publishers, 1974.

Anderson, Susanne, *Song of the Earth Spirit*. San Francisco: Friends of the Earth, 1972.

Arms, Suzanne, *Immaculate Deception*. Houghton Micklin, 1975.

Baker, Dr. Douglas, *Esoteric Anatomy*, Vol. 7 of *The Seven Pillars of Ancient Wisdom*. Little Elephant, Essendon Herts, England, 1976.

Balls, Edward K., *Early Uses of California Plants*. University of California Press, 1972.

Baynes, *The I Ching or Book of Changes*, 1950.

Bean, Constance, *Methods of Childbirth*. Doubleday, 1972.

Beckett, Sarah, *Herbs for Feminine Ailments*. England: Thorsons Publishers

Berends, Berrien Polly, *Whole Parent, Whole Child*. Harper & Row, 1975.

Berlandier, Jean Louis, *The Indians of Texas in 1830*. Washington: Smithsonian Institute Press, 1969.

Bieler, H.G., *Natural Way to Sexual Health*. Charles Publications, 1972.

Food is your Best Medicine. Neville Spearman Ltd., 112 Whitefield St., London, W.I., 1968.

Billings, Dr. John, *The Ovulation Method*. Many editions.

Bing, Elizabeth, *Six Practical Lessons for an Easier Childbirth*.

Bly, Robert, "I Came Out of the Mother Naked", *East West Journal*, August, 1976.

Boston Women's Health Collective, *Our Bodies OurSelves*, 1971. (Recommended as an example of medical/feminist health - I don't agree, however, with the mainly negative reportings of pregnancy, birth and nursing).

Bradley, Robert A., *Husband-Coached Childbirth*. Harper & Row, 1965.

Bragg, Paul, *Preparing for Motherhood, Nature's Way*, Health Science, 1970.

Brennan, Steven F., *Yoga & Medicine*. The Julian Press Inc., 1972.

Brenneman, Helen, **Meditations for the Expectant Mother**, Harold Press, 1968.

Bricklin, Alice, **Motherlove**. Running Tree Press, 1976.

Chertok, Leon, **Motherhood and Personality**. Tavistock Publications, 1969.

Cottrell, Edith Young, **Oats, Peas, Beans and Barley Cookbook**. Woodbridge Press, 1974; P.O. Box 6189, Santa Barbara, CA. 93111.

Cuero, Delfina, **The Autobiography of Delfina Cuero**. Malki Museum Press, 1970.

Culpepper, Nicholas, **Complete Herbal**. London, 1652.

Curtis, Edward S., **The North American Indian**, Vol. 1 & 17. New York: Johnson Reprint Corp., 1970; 111 Fifth Avenue, New York, NY, 10003.

Davis, Adelle, **Let's Have Healthy Children**. Signet, 1972.

Denig, Edwin Thompson, **Five Indian Tribes of the Upper Missouri**. University of Oklahoma Press, 1961.

Diner, Helen, **Mothers & Amazons**. Anchor Books, 1973.

Eiger, Marvin and Sally Olds, **The Complete Book of Breastfeeding**. Bantam Books, 1972.

Ehrenreich, Barbara and Deirdre English, **Complaints & Disorders**. Glass Mountain Pamphlet, 1974.

. **Witches, Midwives & Nurses**. The Feminist Press, 1973.

Ehret, Arnold, **Mucusless Diet Healing System**. Ehret Literature Publishing Co., 1922.

Emergence Publications, **Avoid or Achieve Pregnancy**, 1976.

Ewald, Ellen Buchman, **Recipes For a Small Planet**. Ballantine Books, 1973.

Fallaci, Orianna, **Letter to a Child Never Born**. Simon & Schuster, 1977.

Flanagan, Geraldine, **The First Nine Months of Life**, 1962.

Gabriel, Ingrid, **Herb Identification Handbook**. New York: Sterling Publication Co., Inc.

Gandhi, Mahatma, **Through Self-Control**. India, 1964.

Gauquelinm, Michel, **The Scientific Basis of Astrology**, 1969.

Gerard, **Please Breastfeed Your Baby**. Signet, 1970.

Gladstar, Rosemary, **Country Women's Herbal Handbook**, 1979

Glas, Norbert, M.D., **Conception, Birth & Early Childhood**, Anthroposophic Press, Inc.

Greer, Germaine, **The Female Eunuch**, 1970.

Grieves, Mrs., **The Modern Herbal** (in two volumes). Dover Books.

Harding, Ester M., **Woman's Mysteries**. G. Putnam & Sons, 1971.

Hari Das, Baba(ji). **Between Pleasure & Pain: The Way of Conscious Living**. Sumas: Dharma Sara Publications, 1976; P.O. Box 247, Sumas, Washington, 98295.

Silence Speaks, Sri Rama Foundation, 1977.

The Yellow Book, The Lama Foundation.

Hazell, Lester, **Birth Goes Home**, *1974.*

. **Commonsense Childbirth**, *1969.*

Herbalist Magazine, The *, 224 Draper Lane, P.O. Box 62, Provo, Utah, 84601*

Hermann, Matthias, **Herbs and Medicinal Flowers.** *Galahad Books, 1973.*

Hillman, James, **The Myth of Analysis.** *Northwestern University Press, 1972.*

. **Revisioning Psychology.** *Harper & Row, 1975.*

Hedlicka, Ales, **Physiological and Medicinal Observations Among the Indians of Southwestern United States and Northern Mexico.** *Washington Government Printing Office, 1908*

Hunter, Beatrice Trum, **The Natural Foods Cookbook.** *New York: Pyramid Books, 1961.*

Jackson, Mildred and Terri Teague, **The Handbook of Alternatives to Chemical Medicine.** *Oakland: Lawton-Teague Publications, 1975; P.O. Box 656, Oakland, CA. 94604.*

Janov, Arthur, **The Feeling Child.** *Random House, 1973.*

Jones, David E., **Sanapia, Comanche Medicine Woman.** *San Francisco: Holt, Rinehart, and Winston, 1972.*

Karmel, Marjorie, **Thank You, Dr. Lamaze.** *Doubleday, 1959.*

Kelso, Isa Andeson, **The Causes and Treatment of Women's Ailments,** *from the Self-Help Series. Thorson's Publisher's Limited, 1958.*

Kippley, John, **The Art of Natural Family Planning.** *1975.* Kippley, Sheila, **Breastfeeding and Natural Child Spacing**

Kirk, Donald R., **Wild Edible Plants of the Western United States.** *Naturegraph Publishers, 1970.*

Kitzinger, Sheila, **An Approach to Antenatal Teaching.** *National Childbirth Trust, 1969.*

. **Giving Birth: The Parent's Emotions in Childbirth.** *Taplinger, 1971.*

. **Episiotomy,** *National Childbirth Trust.*

. **The Experience of Childbirth.** *Pelicna, 1967.*

Kloss, Jethro, **Back to Eden.** *Lifeline Books, 1975.*

Koestler, Arthur, **The Roots of Coincidence.** *Random House, 1972.*

Kulvinkas, Victoras, **Love Your Body.** *Omangod Press, 1975; P.O. Box 255, Wethersfield, Connecticut, 06109.*

. **Survival in the 21st Century.** *Omangod Press, 1975.*

Lacey, Louise, **Lunaception,** *1976.*

La Leche League, **The Womanly Art of Breastfeeding,** *1958.*

Lang, Raven, **Birth Book.** *Big Tree Press, 1972.*

"The Politics of Birth at Home", **The Realist,** *February 1972.*

Laszlo, Dr. and Henshaw, **Plant Materials Used by Primitive Peoples to Affect Fertility.**

Le Boyer, Frederick, **Birth Without Violence.** Knopf, 1975.

   . **Loving Hands,** 1976.

Levy, Juliet de Bairch, **Nature's Children.** New York, 1970.

   . **Common Herbs for Natural Health.** Schocken Books, 1966.

Lloyd, J. William, **The Karezza Method,** 1931.

Loewenfeld, Claire, **Herbs, Health, and Cookery.** Hawthorn Books, 1967.

Lurie, Nancy Oestrich (ed.), **Mountain Wolf Woman, Sister of Crashing Thunder.** University of Michigan Press, 1973. Ann Arbor Paperbacks.

Lust, John, **The Herb Book.** Benedict Lust Publications, Box 777. Simi Valley, Ca. 83065

Marion, "Natural Self-Help", **Country Women Magazine,** Issue No. 19. March 1976.

McBride, Angela, **The Growth & Development of Mothers.** Perennial, 1973.

Medvin, Jeannine, **Prenatal Yoga & Natural Birth.** Freestone Publications Collective, 1974.

   . "The Yoga of Conscious Conception", **Yoga Journal.**

Medvin, Michael, **Becoming a Family Joyfully,** Masters Thesis (CSCS), 1975.

   . **On Breastfeeding,** 1971.

Mercante, Anthony S., **The Magic Garden: The Myth and Folklore of Flowers, Plants, Trees, and Herbs.** Harper & Row

Millinaire, Catherine, **Birth.** Harmony Books, 1974.

Montagu, Ashley, **Life Before Birth,** 1964.

   . **Touching,** 1971.

Morgan, Elaine, **The Descent of Woman.**

Mothering (Magazine), Vol. 1; Box 184, Ridgeway, Colorado, 81432.

Muhr, Elaine, **Herbs.**

Muir, Ada, **The Healing Herbs of the Zodiac,** Llewellyn Publications, 1959.

Nelson, Thompson, **Sybil Leek's Book of Herbs.** New York: Nashville Camden Inc.

Neuman, Erich, **The Great Mother,** Bollingen Books.

Newton, Niles, **Maternal Emotions.** Harper & Bros., 1965.

Niethammer, Carolyn, **American Indian Food and Lore.** MacMillan Publishing Co., 1974.

   . **Daughters of the Earth.** Collier Books, 1977.

Nillson, L. and C. Wirsen, **A Child is Born,** 1966.

Nofziger, Margaret, **A Cooperative Method of Natural Birth Control,** The Farm, 1976.

Northecote, Rosalind Lady, **The Book of Herb Lore.** Dover

Oritz, Alfonso, **The Tewa World.** Chicago: University of Chicago Press.

Osawa, George, **Zen Macrobiotics.** The Osawa Foundation, 1965.

Ostrander, Sheila and Lynn Schroeder, **Astrological Birth Control,** 1972.

Our Lady Unique Inclination of the Night, **Cycle One.** Sowing Press, August, 1976; P.O. Box 803, New Brunswick, New Jersey, 18903.

Parsons, Else Clews (ed.), **American Indian Life.** Lincoln: University of Nebraska Press, 1974.

Prentice, T. Merill (watercolors by), **Weeds and Wildflowers of Eastern North America.** Salem: Peabody Museum of Salem, Barre Publications, 1973.

Prensky, Joyce, **Healing Yourself;** 402 15th Avenue E., Seattle, Washington, 98112.

Pryor, Karen, **Nursing Your Baby,**

Psychic Times, "Life Before Life".

Reichard, Gladys A., **Dezba, Woman of the Desert,** Rio Grande Press Inc.; reprent 1971, New Mexico.

Rennie, Susan and Anna Rubin, "Catalog of Resources on Healing", **Chrysalis** (a magazine of women's culture), 1727 N. Spring Street, Los Angeles, California 90012.

Ribble, Margaret, **The Rights of Infants,** Columbia, 1943.

Ritzenhaler, Robert E. and Frederick A. Peterson, **The Mexican Kickapoo Indians.** Greenwood Press, Connecticut, 1970.

Rodale, J.I. and Staff, **Encyclopedia of Organic Gardening and Farming.** Emmaus: Rodale Books Inc., 1970.

Rodale, J.I., **Natural Health & Pregnancy.** Pyramid, 1968.

Rorvik, David, **Your Baby's Sex: Now You Can Choose.** Bantam Books, 1970.

Rose, Jeanne, **Herbs and Things.** Grosset & Dunlap, 1972.

Rosenblum, Art, **Natural Birth Control** (all 4 editions).

Rouse, W.H.D., **Gods, Heroes & Men of Ancient Greece.** A Mentor Book, 1957.

Rush, Anne Kent, **Moon, Moon.** Moonbooks/Random House, 1977.

. **Getting Clear: Female Energy and How to Use It.** Bookworks, 1973.

Rush, Anne Kent and Anica, **Feminism as Therapy,** 1974.

Santee, Ross, **Apache Land.** University of Nebraska Press, 1974.

Scully, Virginia, **A Treasury of American Indian Herbs.** Crown Publishers Inc., 1970.

Shivalila Community, **The Book of the Mother,** 1977. P.O. Box 1441, Bakersfield, CA. 93301.

Smith, Anne M., **Ethnography of the Northern Utes.** Museum of New Mexico Press, 1974.

Sonnichsen, D.L., **The Mescalero Apaches.** University of Oklahoma Press, 1958.

Steiner, Rudolph, **Problems of Nutrition.** Anthroposophic Press Inc., 1969.

Stone, Randolph, **Health Building: The Conscious Art of Living Well.** Ambala, India: Tribune Press, R.R. Sharma, 1963.

Thompson, Dr., **The Improved Family Physician,** *Digest of Midwifery, N.Y. 1833.*

Thompson, Judith, **Healthy Pregnancy the Yoga Way,** *1977.*

Tompkins, Peter and Christopher Bird, **The Secret Life of Plants.** *New York: Avon Books, 1973.*

Urbanowski, Ferris, **Yoga for New Parents,** *Harper's Magazine, 1976.*

Vellay, Pierre, **Childbirth With Confidence.**

Vogel, Virgil J., **American Indian Medicine.** *University of Oklahoma Press, 1970.*

Webster's New World Dictionary, *William Collins & World Pub. Co., Inc. 1975.*

Weideger, Pauline, **Menstruation and Menopause.** *A Delta Book, 1975.*

Well Being Magazine, *833 W. Fir Street, San Diego, California 92101.*

Wesley, John, **Primitive Recipes,** *Woodbridge Press Publishing Co., 1973; P.O. Box 6189, Santa Barbara, CA. 93111.*

White, Ellen G., **Counsels on Diet and Food.** *Review and Herald Publishing Assoc., 1938.*

White, Gregory, **Emergency Childbirth,** *1968.*

Whiting, Alfred F., **Ethnobotany of the Hopi.** *Museum of Northern Arizona, Flagstaff (originally issued in 1939 as Bulletin No. 15).*

Wiener, Michael, **Earth Medicines, Earth Foods.** *Collier Books, 1972.*

Wigmore, Ann, **Be Your Own Doctor.** *Hipprocrates Health Institute.*

World Health Organization, **Cervical Mucus in Human Reproduction,** *1972 Geneva Conference.*

Wright, Erna, **The New Childbirth.** *Tandem Books, 1966.*

Zur Linden, Wilhelm, **A Child is Born.** *Rudolph Steiner Press, 1973.*

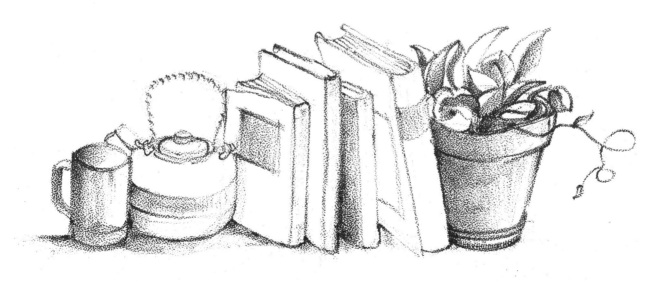

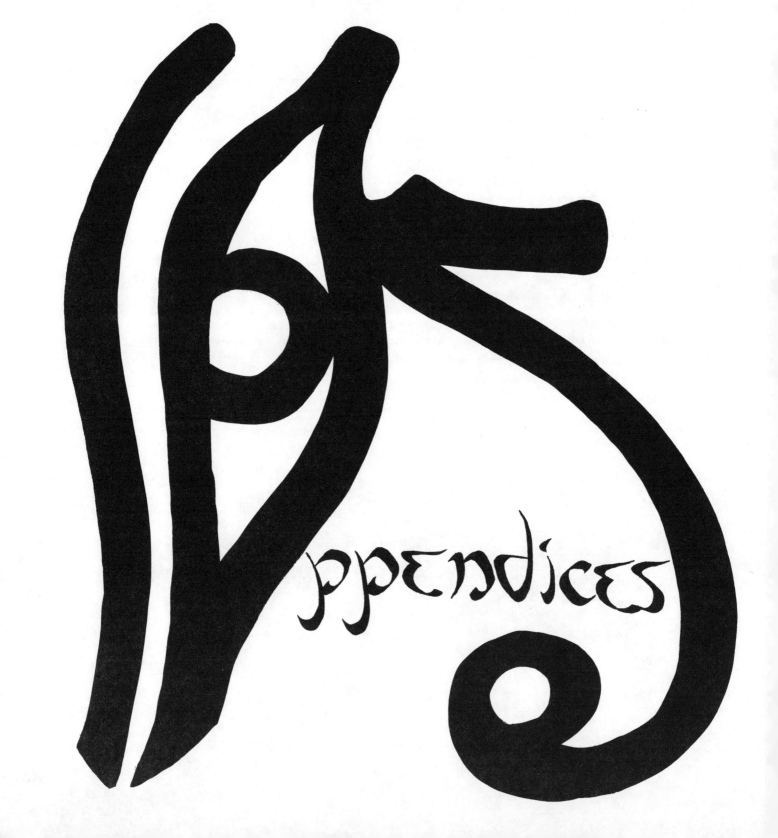

ppendices

Menstrual Poems & Dreams
and a few on weaning

how my period started march 9, 1976

must confess I'd been into the pregnancy drama
ate a grass cookie only three days into the peak
of fertility and opened up to him in the sauna
sperm beings alive in me
reminding me the duty
of hostess and I
reminding them to behave
their impetuous programming
fifty-seven days later and still dry this cunt
like california waiting for rain
carolyn roused out of dream sleepy
song of me being pregnant oh no
yes another baby to contain
to let go of
to learn how to love
to help me
help me wean my toddling twins
help me learn who I am
help me
crazy with my baby need
more of me emerges
sweet woman rising strong
I let him play
delilah to my samson
locks come off
locks come off
looney in cancer
the yoga teacher
within
feels the purification
hears the holy hiss
sound her heart's path
fire-bath
baby shiva burning
baby shiva burning
now I will flow
my choice
cheyenne comes on so tender
curling latching on

kitten-lipped
we melt
milked so purely
I begin to bleed
indeed
more of me emerges
sweet woman rising strong
"death ripens noiselessly inside of me"
An egg of ashes
drops from Eden
whitening the love -
nest
Sounding
cilia applause
(cosmos lined up
along the tubes)
tiding a monthly hope
towards home
"Whipping passion up
into poetry"
the seed grows
through the earth
but not rooted
to mother
and I bleed
another poem
while off the wheel
for awhile
awaiting
the red
"day 65 of my breastfeeding-menstrual cycle"
Cervix feels of the sea
anenome
imagine squid mouthed
muscle prayers
the blood of virgin mary
is actually the salt
of the sea
tears of primordial grief
ocean grave for another ovum
menstrual current
my womb is a tomb
a motel host
for the transient dead
the ocean receives
all the dead
menstrual current

Three years since the tidings of my womb
red contractions
earth's sanguine tears
embrace me as an old friend

Jeannine Parvati's Dreams
Ovulation Dreams

When I first began paying attention to my possible times of fertility, I dreamed the following:

". . . . I walk into the kitchen, open the refrigerator, and eggs fall out."

This was part of a very long dream and if I hadn't bothered to write it down, the most important passage might have been left unrealized. The kitchen is my symbol of nourishment; a refrigerator, that which contains and keeps from spoiling the food, or raw material of living. I keep this energy in the cooler around at this time in my life when approaching ovulation, I do not want more babies, so I store my hot stuff away. But I open the frigidaire (dare I be frigid) to see my eggs fall out - or ovulate. Sure enough, I check out my cervical mucus, and it had changed from the creamy fertile mucus to spinnbarkeit, clear stringy mucus signaling the ovulation is imminent, or has just occurred. I posit that ovulation had just occurred in the night, probably when I was dreaming about the eggs falling out. The body and her dreams can exist side by side with our waking "reality" - we need not try to get something out of dreams while awake - the messages, when we are ready to hear them, will make them-selves felt and understood.

Another, less obvious, ovulation dream: August 12, 1977 - Moon in Leo (My natal moon sign!)

"I am midwiving. A baby is born whom I catch - again, rush of ecstasy as we welcome this new being to our planet. I look around for something sterile with which to cut loose this baby. When the husband eventually cuts the cord, and the need for something sterile is imminent, I do the best with what we have, but there's nothing sterile. Tie the babe off with a shoe lace - but the stump begins to swell, so I untie the cord and a light pink fluid flows out. Again, no sterile string to finish off the birthing process. We use what's available but I watch closely for any signs of backing up, infections or pressure. The birthing family is beautiful, and I, as usual am in love with the baby.

Here I am deeply exploring a decision not to have more babies now in my life. Michael and I are attentive to our fertility cycle, and when the sexual energy swells up, we look for something to tell us that we are infertile (sterile).

Menstrual Dream

This reflects my waking world beliefs about bleeding and child-tending at the same time:

Day 2 of my period. Moon in Capricorn.

"Tami and I are living together and agreeing that when she is working, I take care of the children. I ask her help in cleaning the house saying that if my work is of equal value, i.e. caring for the children, to her art work,

then we should both bear equal responsibility for cleaning the house daily. I didn't want to have to take care of kids and clean house at the same time. She agrees."

When we've lost our traditions, we got to start somewhere. Traditionally, women of this continent, the American Indians, would do their internal "housecleaning" or menstruation apart from the responsibilities of childcare. We, as mothers, often become irritable at our young while in our moon. And it is because we need time to mother ourselves now, for just two days or so, each month. Let's re-instate this tradition - asking time off from work, babysitting one another's children, and giving ourselves back our roots.

Of course we **can** take care of worldly tasks, our children and homes, and even out-in-the-world businesses, but the question is, do we want to? Most women I know enjoy the pacing and rhythm of monthly vacations, inside and out.

My friend Betty Hudleston and I enjoy viewing our menses as clearing us to be the receptive saviours of our evolving species - it's hard to remain convinced of this when confronting male energy every day of the year!

Ovulation Dream

JUNE 11, 1977, Day 18, Moon in Aries. Spinnbarkeit mucus.

"Walk through a dark neighborhood just as an old man calls me - I am a little afraid and excited. Walk through several groups of men and then see my daughter Loi. I run to her, hug her - saying her name with great love over and over. She smiles and as I am saying "We're home!", I realize **she's** home and we're visiting together out of our bodies. I say this to her aloud, realizing that I am lucid, i.e. aware that I am dreaming yet still in the dream. I begin to feel the familiar streaming of energy, like a whirlwind inside, and then the thought, "I want to fly to God" carries me up and up. Delightful sensation of dissolution. Awake exhilarated and happy."

Flying dreams, lucid dreams, out of the ordinary experiences are more common I have found, in review of my eight years of dream journals, during the ovulation time of the woman's cycle. Many researchers have validated the presence of male figures in ovulatory dreams also.

The night before this dream, I had checked my own cervix during a dream to discover spinnbarkeitt mucus. Sure enough, I woke and then inserted my fingers into my cunt to feel a sample of long stringy cervical mucus. At this time in my life, I'd always be surprised by ovulation as my nursing three year old twins played havoc with my hormones. The more I nursed, the less often I would ovulate, and so on. . .

Dreams began to visit me, as healers, when I ceased probing and policing them for signs of returning fertility. A good example of how the internal **is** the external is my policeman story. During one time in my life, when my relationship to love was all absorbing, knowing for sure exactly when I was fertile meant my very own survival.

*Or so it seemed. I was enjoying many sperm visitors in me, yet my own two babies were yet a year. Clearly, I didn't need more babies, not now. So I could 1) give up sex, 2) remain infertile or 3) pinpoint the exact time of fertility and avoid my friends the sperm, around that phase. No cycle, I was nursing **full** time. At one point, I figured out that I gave more milk than our prize family goat. In any case, I chose to be quite vigilant about any sign of fertility. My body became a vehicle for my search. Daily I checked basal body temperature. I checked my mucus. I searched my dreams and policed my fantasies. I drank my herbal blends to give me enough energy to do all this. The funny thing was, I was always being stopped by the police when I drove the car for vehicle violations. Me, who in eleven years of perfect driving, was now being cited daily for some infraction or the other. The tail light went out - so I paid more attention to the color of my own bottom and began sunbathing again - then the exhaust valve broke off, so I stopped smoking - and so on. The point of this story is that as soon as I stopped policing my being for these signals of fertility, I was able to drive safely without any more vehicle inspections from the police. That meant my dreams too. If some mornings, they preferred to hide, that was okay. The invitation remained open all day and sometimes one dream or two would whisper to me as I went about my work. Like the book that falls open to a word which restimulates a dream sequence. Or the person who comes unexpectedly bringing with her an image from last night's dream. Little ways to re-own pieces of one's life, living as metaphor, as Iris.*

Dream the day before menstruation, December 8, 1976. Moon in Cancer.
"Home and the space is changing. I say I prefer children living here rather than an empty house. Then I add that I wanted to have another baby but now that there's not a supportive community to help me, I won't get pregnant."

Awake to my menstrual flow. House is body, cleaning the purification of menstruation. I do want to contain more children, but not until my community is more supportive. It's not uncommon to have clear messages in my dreams, if I posit my need clearly.

Another Typical Ovulation Dream

FEBRUARY 24, 1977. Moon in Taurus, Day 76.

"On a beach with lots of dancers. We all hold hands and run and dance on the sand. We sit down and listen to a pregnant couple talk about their emotional lability. I am responsive to them and tell them about the anant vayu (a wind which inhabits women during pregnancy) and then suggest they ask Babaji, who is seated with us. Perhaps he'll say when it leaves after birthing. A group of dancers go into a big hall. They're about to do a folk dance. I run there, looking/hoping to find a partner. The first that could possible be my partner is attractive, but I let him pass on by."

The time of ovulation is the opportunity for pregnancy. I let my partner in this dance pass on by. I feel the rush of progesterone in my body and see a pregnant couple as a way to work out the surge of moods that come at this time. Babaji is my highest yogi-self, and he is often in ovulation dreams.

Nadine's Dreams

"So Linda calls you Tit, huh?". Linda has a pen in her hand. I am afraid she will scratch me with it. I hold my thigh. She draws a symbol on my left breast and a small scribble on the right one. Linda's presence flows thru out my being. I experience her as a shaman. Her words to me are unquestioned truth. There are comfrey plants around us.

The following night I ask my dreams what the symbol means. I dream - A drawing of Indian female bodies that range from infant, young girl, adult woman, pregnant woman and an old woman. They are standing in a line and there is a symbol under each one. The pregnant woman has the identical marking that Linda had drawn on my breast the night before.

Later that month I learn that I am pregnant and have an abortion.

Ovulation Dreams

There's a lush garden growing with a tomato tree in the center. A fence surrounds the garden. Jokingly I race two men to the tomatoes. I run thru an open gate and manage to get there before them. There is a young woman driving a light blue volks. She is looking for a place to park the car where it will be safe.
In all seriousness, I am racing to get to my egg before they are made fertile by the men. The volks, the light blue color, indicates again the egg in its state of ovulation.

I plant an apple tree and in a relatively short time it has grown quite big, is firmly rooted and bearing fruit. I hope its not too close to the "cedar" tree and has room to grow.

This dream reveals a message to me about my physical and emotional state in relation to my lover. The "cedar", seeder needs to be a sufficient distance away in order that I don't become implanted with his seeds and so that I have space to grow, spread my own roots.

I am driving along and a Construction Man holds up a Stop sign.

Stop baby construction by limiting intercourse for now.

Two lines of virgins form an isle. A woman draped in veils walks step by step down the center. When she

gets to the end where no more are standing, a second woman approaches with a sword and cuts thru the other woman's veils. She slices her back, face, and chest. "You have failed. You had no guard, no protection, no tradition or basis for your movements. It was shallow and meaningless.
Now it is my turn. I choose to walk upon an unlevel, slightly twisted sheet of metal. I walk barefoot. The woman comes toward me with her sword, but I duck and sway. I arch as if going under a limbo stick - moving down the isle. There is no groom. I marry myself.

Then the woman walks down a path with me. I am wearing my mother's bright green spring coat. "You dress immaturely, but that's okay, my lover also dresses like that, I sort of like it." At the end of our walk there is a beautiful wild flower that I feel extremely intimate and connected with.

April 14, 1974 Menstrual Dream

A woman takes me to her room and shows me her menstrual blood. She said she saves it from her first period and intends to feed it to her first baby and didn't want to throw it out. I say mine has returned to the earth.

April 25, 1974

I'm walking with Arnell. We are reading a story together. Walking in a green field with flowers, then suddenly I get an urge and drop the book and run. I run fast and long but my legs don't feel tired. I feel like I could keep on going. I feel my body raise and I AM FLYING. I hear flapping, like wings, the air rushes around me. I feel like there's someway else I can use this power. I wake.

November 5, 1973 Menstrual Dream

"I'm at a grocery store with my sister, Adrienne. She's not feeling well and tries to think of a way to get home. As I wait I write in my journal - the key words are "Twins". Everywhere I look there seems to be a large and then its miniature identical. There are several pairs of brothers and sisters. One small boy draws a cartoon character for another child.

I get in my car to take Adrienne home. I bring a blanket. Inside there are many different colored fish. We drive for a while and then stop at a cliff overlooking the ocean. Its an extremely breathtaking view. We sit on the sand dunes, which bear strange mosaic patterns as if one were seeing it stoned. There is some reference made about a cocaine culture once living here. Also, an agreement about if you have your house evaluated then anyone after that is allowed inside, even if you don't want them to.

We leave the sand dunes and follow a path that leads to a small island. There is shallow water around it that large peacock birds are wading in and drinking. The colors in the dream now become very intense. The birds' tail feathers are spread wide revealing irredescent blues and purples, their eyes are large. The island is carpeted with emerald green moss. Very few people are ever allowed to cross over to its shore. I ask Alan what the name of the place is. I say there's a place in Connecticut, (the state I was born) called Deadman's Gulch. Alan calls it Paradise Isle. It's very tropical looking covered with thick greenery and blossoms. I cross the water alone and step onto the island. I notice a woman dressed in uniform behind a rock. I've never seen her before but in the dream she's from my self defense class. The woman is holding a rifle and as she thrusts it forward she knocks a bird in her way. She approaches me. Then I notice to my left a young beautiful woman dressed in flowers - red roses and lush green petals. She lies down with her arms across her chest like she's preparing to die. Her little girl and dog run towards her but she motions them to return. "I am sorry dear but it is time for me to go." I awake with strong feelings of power."

This dream has been one of the most significant of my life. I believe this menstruation marked a letting go of a naive self. Its blood carried away a youthful dependency, allowing for a stronger, more responsible, and assertive self to surface. It marks an initiation rite, a death and a letting go in order that a new birth may take place, evolving from a child to a mature woman.

Meditations for Conception

"Parents should listen inwardly, in order to hear the call, to discover when their child will come to them. They will only find out if they can hear the call. But frequently it happens under present day conditions, the more delicate feelings cannot awaken in the soul. . . it has become usual to fix the time for the coming of children according to practical ideas; whether the man has a big enough income, and so forth."[1] - Norbert Glas, M.D.

Meditation practice can be of great value not only in fertility awareness but obviously in all areas of experience. The mindfulness developed by meditation brings clarity to some larger - than - self issues about the nature of attachment. Babies, literally, are females' greatest attachments.

Pregnancy affords to the woman the opportunity to contain the Other, Beloved Thou - Women thusly are able to know the experience of being-within **and** being-the-one-who-contains-within. It is an easy way to achieve "oneness" with another - be their mama.

By insighting, I trip upon this fear of giving birth to a baby who one day in turn asks contemptuously why I brought him to this planet in the first place? Long periods of attention to **avoidance** of pregnancy creates fantasies such as these. It is a hazard well worth the risk, uncovering of fearful energy that binds the life-force and breath of my being. The more I'm aware of charged thoughts and the feeling indelibly with them, the less I need act them out unconsciously. The place to read these scripts for parenthood are often best found in dreams. Meditation on dreams, an inward moving process that produces sensations much like the hormones of pregnancy.

"In ancient times, the mother was deeply connected with the coming child, even before conception. She lived in a dream-like world and experienced much of the supersensible realm in her feeling life."[2] - Glas

Meditations on the Egg Self

"Eggs correspond to the original void source."
"The egg is synonymous with the heart center of the body."
"It all begins humming, in the egg."
Egg on my beard - egg you on - egg/head - nest/egg -
Nksuano - the Moon-Egg of China
The Orphic Egg
    of the alchemists
The Easter Egg
    of the Christians
The Druidic Egg
    of the world

*Eggs are the seeds - they represent hope. In women, all of the eggs needed in one's life-time are born within; awaiting ripening. Men may be able to produce their seed, the sperm, every three days. Perhaps men have cycles of fertility also - and our verifying certain aspects of fertility awareness and behavior on the assumption that each and every ejaculation contains impregnating sperm is invalid. Men are more fertile around their birthdays and every four months thereafter, is one myth and bio-rhythms could be a useful tool in our home science. Meditation makes the subtle cycles of reality a bit clearer. The image of the WHEEL from Buddhism is metaphorically ideal for female sexuality - with the menstrual cycles, eggs, and circle of secrets about birth and death. My favorite meditation is listening to the circle of breath - ajapna mantram it is called - just being aware of the sound of your own breath. The sound of the newborn's first breath - fresh from God. Sometimes in meditation it is as if the Goddess were **breathing** me!*

*The Madonna is the ideal upon which to meditate while pregnant - she symbolizes the calling down from the heavens the spirit into the child, and the compassionate motherlove evoked in service to God. However, when not into conceiving or mothering, the image of Artemis, Diana (the Moon - goddess of the hunt and the dance of fertility) is more appropos. She is the twin of Apollo and master of the bow as well. Contemplation of Her results sometimes in a feeling for the wildness in birthing and a healthy respect for the process. Her mother Leto held onto a palm tree and the earth shook with joy when her brother was born. She will reveal herself to women - but if we are Actaeon-like in our seeking, and come upon this goddess unprepared, we may suffer the same fate, hounded by self-doubts and our own **haunting thoughts**.*

*Meditation creates a space for the community within to get to know one another. From my meditations two important leaders have emerged - they're representational of my two strongest voices in the fertility choir. The Madonna - and the Feminist: the mother of the lord and the mother of my Self. The one who only serves and the one who is learning how to fully desire. "There isn't anything yet I've found to be as holy as mothering." Meditation allows glimpses into **just being** that is "as holy" as being a mother, or lover - for that matter. Ephesus, the many-breasted one and birth-goddess is a melting of the two for me. * Tarot meditations are a great tool -*

they can be used specifically, and topically by asking simple questions to the divinatory element in the reading or deeper insights come from sitting in silence with the image of a particular card for long periods of time. I ask the Empress if I am fertile or not in meditations. If she speaks to me, I figure that I am very fecund. Yet it is the High Priestess who draws me lately from the deck. And before her, I am humble.

*Not only does this goddess love her sex but all aspects of femininity - and to such an extreme of sprouting many breasts over her trunk. My approach to mothering has been a lot like this and my enjoyment of breastfeeding is such that I call the experience orgasmic. The tit is the external placenta continuing the nourishing and psychic link between baby and mother. Sometimes I feel like my entire trunk is flowing with the sweet nectar, just like Ephesus.

FOOTNOTES

1. **Conception, Birth and Early Childhood** by Norbert Glas, M.D. Anthroposophic Press, Inc. 258 Hungry Hollow Road, Spring Valley, N.Y. 10977, 1972, P. 7.

2. IBID, P. 4

To Conceive or Not To Conceive:
Problems with Conception, Miscarriages, & Still Births
~Marcia Starck

While most of today's women are trying every possible form of birth control to avoid conception, there are still a handful who are desperately attempting to conceive. Medical Astrology can be of assistance in showing what the difficulties are and what time periods might be the best for these women. I have studied many of these charts and have been specifically working with eight of these women.

Some women who are born at new and full moons have more trouble conceiving than other moon phases, and once they do conceive, may have problems carrying the child. They are more prone to miscarriages than other soli-lunar types. Next in line are those born during the first and last quarter (in other words, sun squaring moon).

In terms of the general pattern of the chart, Libra is the most commonly found Ascendant, which usually places Aquarius on the fifth house cusp. Aquarius is a fairly barren sign and may indicate either no children or an adopted child at some point in the life. Planets occupying the fifth house would of course alter this. In one of the eight charts, a woman with Aquarius on her fifth and Venus in it, had not been able to conceive until her 37th year, when Uranus squared her fifth house Venus, and she unexpectedly became pregnant.

Aspects to the moon should be considered in determining a woman's fertility and the difficulties she may encounter during pregnancy. Hard aspects can indicate more problems, and it will be important for the woman to watch her health carefully. The most important aspects to consider are Moon to Mars and Moon to Pluto. Hard aspects to both of these planets may indicate problems during pregnancy or a difficult delivery with excessive hemorrhage, particularly if Mars is involved. Most of my example charts have hard aspects to both Mars and Pluto. Those women who have had mis-carriages or still births usually have the Pluto aspect.

Hard aspects from Saturn to the Moon are found in cases where the woman has never been able to conceive.· Uranus and Neptune causing hard aspects to the Moon don't seem to be too prevalent in this group. Two women have the Uranus and two the Neptune. Uranus aspects would have to do with unexpected pregnancy, and in the case of the 37 year old who had never conceived, Uranus is opposite her Moon. Hard aspects to Neptune may have to do with the illusion of wanting to have a child where it is not practically feasible. In example No. 1, Moon is broadly conjunct Neptune. This woman had no difficulty conceiving her first child, but now there is some question as to whether her husband wants another child (she **thinks** she does), so she has not been able to conceive.

Having surveyed the general chart indicators, it is helpful to look at a few midpoints to get the full picture. The three midpoints which have particular relevance in these cases are Moon/Venus, which is the female ability to conceive; Moon/Mars having to do with sexual problems, pregnancies, and abortions; and Venus/Mars, menstruation difficulties and sexual problems.

For purposes of general health, Saturn/Neptune, the basic health axis, Mars/Saturn, the body structure, and Mars/Neptune, susceptibility to infections and toxins, should also be computed. (In determining midpoints, 8 midpoints are used. For example, if the midpoint comes out to be 15 Libra, then 15 degrees of all the cardinal signs would be involved, as well as the indirect midpoints, which are 45° away - thus 0 of the mutable signs).

In half of these cases, the Moon/Venus midpoint equals Neptune which, according to Ebertin, indicates weakened or abnormal glandular activity. Usually abnormal glandular activity is related to emotional disturbances either in this lifetime or in past ones. Moon/Venus = Neptune may also indicate illusions about conception. In several other cases, Moon/Venus midpoint =

Saturn which can be inhibited glandular activity and often is related to a malfunctioning thyroid. A few of these women have been given thyroid supplements by their doctors, which have proved helpful. With the Moon/Mars and Venus/Mars midpoints, the charts in which they equal Pluto is where there have been cases of mis-carriage or still-birth.

Checking out the general health midpoints, the most significant pattern is the Saturn/Neptune midpoint = Mercury. This shows that many of these women have problems with their nervous system, and that worry and anxiety may have much to do with their inability to conceive.

Now, what measures can be taken to help some of these women so that they might bear children? Exercise can be very helpful, especially yoga postures since they relax and stretch the internal organs. In the case of the woman who did not conceive until the age of 37, she had recently started jogging. This was the only new addition to her regime.

Changes in diet, as well as vitamin and mineral supplements, have played an important part. In several of these women the thyroid gland was found to be under-active. The use of kelp and other iodine sources have restored it to normal functioning. Others have been strongly lacking calcium and magnesium. They found that when increasing their calcium and magnesium intake through foods, as well as through mineral supplements and cell salts, their general health as well as the condition of their nervous system improved. All of the cases found a strong B-complex to be of much help in eliminating their anxieties and worries.

In aiding these women to find particularly fertile periods, transits through the fifth house should be checked, as well as progressed aspects to the ruler of the fifth. Planets activating the Moon/Venus midpoints, especially Sun, Venus and Jupiter, could indicate a particularly fertile time. Transits of Pluto or Neptune over some of the heavy planets should be avoided as they often indicate hidden changes. New Moon, full Moon, and first and last quarter types should conceive during their ovulation period rather than during their cosmic fertility cycle to avoid difficulties.

The Mother of Plants ～THE MOON

The moon and herbs and women have been connected throughout the ages. Pliny said, "The moon saturates the earth with water and by its approach (becoming fuller, waxing) fills bodies, while by its departure it empties them". **The moon is the planet of breath and soul.** More than one animistic culture has believed that it is the moon which impregnates women. And harvesting at the full moon has been suggested by many peoples - especially herbs and other fruits of the earth, like babies. Samuel Deane (1733 - 1814) said, "... as we know both animals and vegetables are influenced by the moon in some cases, why may we not suppose a greater quantity of spirit is sent up into the fruit, when the attraction of the heavenly bodies is greatest".

There is a lot more to be said about growing your herbs, gathering them respectfully in the "bush" - plus being aware of the effects of the moon and other heavenly bodies upon our women's bodies/psyches. And we will say it; next book on Conscious Conception.

As the moon is but one luminary in the heavens associated with plants and women, a brief look at the science of astrology and how it applies to herbs is paramount. As in all sciences, serious study is needed in order to "speak the language". It is beyond the scope of this book to introduce the novice into the elegant world of astrology, **whose practice brings meaning to our lives.** Astrology moves me in circles; it is yet another tool of the gods and goddesses, or forces, to be understood cyclically and in definite rhythms.

Gail Walker, in "Moon Changes" writes, "Women's bodies cycle. The connection between women's physical nature and the moon changes was made long ago. The moon was presumed to be the fertilizing force that impregnated women. It was said that the light of the full moon upon a woman's naked belly caused her to be with child.

It may be that male's fascination with the full moon reveals an attempt to connect with their own cyclic nature. It is, perhaps, by projection onto the full moon that men come closest to a tangible understanding of a seemingly feminine cycling", - from **Lady Unique Inclination of the Night**.Cycle I.

The plants, too, are governed by the movement of planets. You can observe this for yourself by making good friends with an herb and then being with her in the morning, when the **solar force** comes on, and then in the evening during the reign of that queen-of-night, our earthly **moon**. She will feel different - for one, respiration is reversed from night to day in a plant. There are also some subtle changes occurring through various transits of planets daily, monthly, and yearly. An obvious example of this is how the sunflower is at its zenith during the time that the sun is in the zodiacal constellation of Leo. Or how Lady Slipper, traditionally used to calm hysteria, feels so soothing during the Aquarian time of the year.

Popular astrology has limited our understanding by focusing only on the Sun **sign** of an individual. What else can one expect in a **patriarchy**? Where is the attention to the Moon? I identify with my lunar placement so deeply because I am a woman. Most astrologers (with the exception of Dane Rudhyar - read **Rania**) are writing from the masculine conception of the universe. A feminine cosmology would not have newspaper columns in adoration of but one force within. The sun sign is only your birthday. Astrological study brings many more re-births. And so it is when we are working with herbs that the entire map of a person, their horoscope, is taken into account (and I might add to look at transits and progressions, and midpoints, also!). The **rising sign**, only known when the moment of the individual's first breath was taken (at birth), is needed to see the natal constitution. Herbs that are in harmony with the rising sign then are indicated first.

Ada Muir, in **The Healing Signs of the Zodiac**, gives an excellent and simple introduction to what could be a complicated study. For example: a woman suffering by obsessive sexual desires, usually has a venus-uranus affliction either by transit, progression or natally (meaning quickly, has been building up to, and/or, all the time). The sexual excesses can be helped by the herb Southernwood, acting as a tonic. And there is a science to choosing the remedy - medical astrology has much to offer any herbalist or healer.

*Southernwood, by the way, is commonly called "Old Man" - the slang term meaning **my mate** by many new-age (aquarian-uranian) women. Traditionally it's been used to treat hysteria.*

*One idea the good Doctor Astrology and I enjoyed many moons ago was the creation of a zodiacal flower and herb garden. A mandala of color and scent reflecting one's natal horoscope - with a bed of chamomile to lay upon in the center. Exquisite star perennials could be placed in the various houses of herbs as representations of planets. You could watch bees pollinate the planets, their path of flight describing the aspects between the forces within your Self. Sitting in a circle of friends. Geocentric and grounded: with the delight of the heavens surrounding. One summer when the babies were small, I used to meditate in the center of a garden such as that. Towards the end of that sunny practice, the flowers had grown right toward the center of the meditation area - which was a plywood platform on the earth covered with a yoga mat, and many hours of surrendering. It was quite beautiful to see plants spiraling toward me during morning sadhana, some even growing **horizontal** toward the yoga space.*

The planets are symbols for forces working within us; the images are the gods and goddesses, and the whole human experience becomes a mandala of meditation. Astrology can give us back our souls.

And when we bring soul-force with us in herbology, the science becomes an art. This, is healing.

Pregnancy & Childbirth, Nature's Way
~Rosemary Sutton

"Nothing is so beautiful as a ship at full sail, or a woman great with child."

When a woman is pregnant and "great with child", she feels, with deep heart's instinct, her oneness with the flow of creation, the birth/death cycle. Divine Mother sends her gifts of guidance to her daughters: the strengthening and healing herbs, grasses, and flowers. Almost half-remembered in their use.

Tonic teas should be drunk throughout pregnancy, to insure an easy birthing. Raspberry leaf tea is the tried and true tonic to the uterus, as are squaw vine and wild yam root. For the unsettled stomach, which is sometimes felt in the early months, teas of fennel leaf or seed, wild yam root, mint, or a pinch of golden seal is in order.

Nutritional requirements are high during pregnancy. Calcium is essential for bone and tooth formation; good sources are salads of amaranth, borage, comfrey, coriander, dandelion, mustard greens, and watercress. Iron is found in these too, and in chives and burdock root. Folic acid is abundant in all leafy greens.

Begin early to condition the skin, preparing for smooth stretching. Add a strong tea of comfrey leaf or root to the bath, or take as a sitz bath. After bathing, body oil is helpful to lubricate the skin and maintain its elasticity. An oil I like is made by **gently** heating together 2 cups of oil (olive, sesame, almond, or the like) with a handful each of elder blossoms and comfrey. Part of the oil could be wheat germ oil or capsules of Vitamin E could be opened and added. The heat of a summer's day, or perhaps two, is enough to steep the oil. After cooling, add finely crushed pollen, an incredible skin builder, and a few drops of a pure essential oil, for the senses.

The perineum, the skin below the vagina, should be conditioned throughout pregnancy with sunlight, fresh air, and massage with the body oil. If it should tear, a poultice of good ole comfrey (fresh, preferably) will be healing.

As your time approaches, have your medicine chest well stocked. Have on hand pennyroyal leaf and oil, tansy, and blue cohosh. These herbs, valued as they are for bringing on a delayed menstrual flow, are not normally called upon in pregnancy. But if you wish to hasten a long labor, or bring on labor when the water has broken but contractions not yet begun, then use these herbs. The scent of the pennyroyal oil would be inhaled, or the oil could be poured in simmering water to vaporize the room. The pennyroyal leaf, tansy, and blue cohosh would be taken as teas.

For normal labor, a gentle relaxant tea of chamomile and catnip flavored with hibiscus flowers, is useful to moisten dry lips and face, and is a delicious celebration drink later.

The little stem of the umbilical cord will usually not need any special care. Comfrey leaves, crushed and wrapped inside a cabbage leaf could be laid across the navel (the origin maybe of the legend of finding the baby under a cabbage?). Indians of this area used mugwort leaves to hasten healing.

Milk will flow in abundance to the mother getting enough rest and good liquids. Fennel tea is a galactgogue: it increases the milk. An old legend says that placing pimpernel roots next to the breasts will cause a copious flow. Sage and parsley tend to dry up the milk.

Remember that the essential oils of herbs, along with garlic and onions, are not, unlike other foods, filtered by the mother's body, but instead pass directly into her milk. The babe then receives the benefits and effects of all herbs the mother ingests. So if your colicky child refuses chamomile tea (though few will!), drink large amounts yourself and rest assured.

For sore nipples, mix the body oil with pure lanolin and rub in. If a breast infection develops, drink echinacea tea and take *golden seal* and *myrrh gum capsules, as natural antibiotics. Hot poultices of potato, or alternate hot & cold applications of cloths wrung out in tea will give relief.*

Bathing is a wonderfully relaxing experience after a full day of child care. Add a bit of pine needle essence to your bath to really unwind. To soothe the babe's skin, a gentle infusion of chamomile and bran can be strained and added to the water. Soap can irritate tender skin. If really dirty, the little one can be scrubbed with oatmeal tied in a kerchief. It forms a creamy liquid in water. Be sure to rinse well. Oiling the diaper area with good quality olive oil is a rash preventative.

Ideally, of course, each and everyone should have an herb garden —
perhaps tucked amongst the vegetables and flowers,
or a separate space, to wander in & dream of a babe's sweet face.

On Total Mothering

My sadhana is turning women on to their responsibilities and gift of being their baby's healer. Herbal Infant Care is really woven through this book, but Total Mothering, as a healing process, needs a space of its own.

*Our Center for Family Growth has long been educating families about the caring and tending of their baby's health. This begins before conception, with the mother and father doing all they can towards readying their bodies/psyches for the experience of pregnancy, birthing and lactation. The full expression of this is total parenting - but since this is a book whose readership primarily is for women, the main focus is on total mothering. "Total" means full, deep, complete - there is nothing withheld from your baby - there is present a concern for the welfare of your baby on all levels of reality - not only as a body whose health a mother largely makes or breaks, but to the baby as a soul, spirit, **feeling** being. I've seen babies with **arthritis** - whose parents won't let be angry and **keep the child in a constant state of frustration, hidden by a facade of being the "good baby" who** never makes a fuss. I've seen babies, so-called "good" with the angriest rashes all over their skins. I've seen babies with constant ear infections - a protection from hearing what their environment is telling them, because it doesn't match up with a baby's felt experience. And I've seen babies with "weepy" eye infections - their mamas are the ones that soothe by saying, "Don't cry!" when their babes are in pain. The word is magic - babies are literal creatures and saying to your child with the scraped knee, "You're O.K." when she obviously is hurting. This is not only confusing but dangerous. The best way to avoid a child's illness is to be healthy oneself. Children imitate and your aches and pains set examples. Psychosomatic is an overworked word but does suggest itself here. Seeing positive thought forms of a healthy and beautiful baby will create one. Giving messages to your children like, "You'll catch cold" will also bring this about. You train your children to be sick - by direct and indirect messages and by daily living practices. Look at your own messages about health and choose which are helpful and which are not. "Hereditary" diseases are a good place to begin. In my mother's family it was heart disease. Well, I've had a lot of work to do on this life-script. I bought into it as a baby by manifesting a murmur* and was on my way to being a weak and delicate child til I understood that the lesson here was metaphoric - the physical heart stood for the emotional heart. My practice has been one of learning to love openly and in **rhythm** with the cosmos. Learning the tempo of love is connected with my recovery, and the averting of this serious disease that has carried off most my elder relatives at a young age. Likewise with my constellation of allergies which is discussed elsewhere in the book.*

*Total mothering means that after the birthing of your baby, the oneness is maintained via the breasts as an external placenta. This means that the baby is carried on your body and never far from your titties. There are no pacifiers other than your body, and eventually every mother can learn how to let her milk down only when the baby's need is for nourishment. Other times, when we nurse our babies to soothe them but they're aren't hungry, the let-down reflex is inhibited - this can be brought about by conscious attention (which is learned through any meditative discipline) to **psychically** feeding the needy baby with your juicy loving rahter than gorging them with too much milk.*

*Total mothering means sleeping with your babies/children. Since one third of our lives are spent sleeping, and nursing babies and mothers even have simultaneous dreams, this great portion of the mothering experience is best served in the same bed. Babies are only babies for such a short time - whereas husbands can be babies all their lives - especially if they didn't get their needs satisfied by their own mothers. For mates who resist sleeping with their children, you might add a little of your breast milk to their food, or have them nurse in order to awaken a mothering/fathering instinct. Prolactin, the hormone of mothering **present in breast milk, is so strong when given to roosters they stop crowing and go sit on eggs.** I've never heard of folks rolling over onto sleeping babies - unless drunk. You'll be amazed at how aware you are of your baby as she lays asleep next to you.*

Nightly nursings then become a pleasure when all you have to do is roll over and plop a tit into a hungry mouth. And the real terror of awaking in the middle of the night alone is prevented - most kids with any moxie crawl back into their parent's beds anyway.

*Total mothering means not supplementing your perfect milk with "baby foods". Many allergies and digestive troubles will be avoided by nursing your baby totally and awaiting the sign of teeth before introducing solid or even semi-solid foods. I let my three children actually pick up the food themselves, get it into their mouths, and swallow before I made solid foods available. Once solid foods are introduced, the return of fertility is imminent also. For up til now, when one practices total mothering, your **body** know you have a baby, so there's no need to return to fertility in order to produce another one. Refer to Sheila Kippley's book on **Breast Feeding and Natural Child Spacing** for a fuller discussion of this. And lastly, total mothering means SURRENDER. Our work is as important as any spiritual adept,[1] for when we truly surrender to the needs of our babies, we forget ourselves in the process, just the same way as a yogi forgets himself in meditation. You can make the service of child-care a meditation or a hassle. It's up to you, and our culture, and our emerging mythology. Personally, I won't conceive babies unless the father is into it equally - down to the diapers as well as the support, both emotional as well as physical. But there are many ways to rightously care for babies and the babies, bless them, teach us how if we but listen.*

But how can we meet the needs of our little ones purely when looking from our own unmet ones? Learn to express your feelings and fill your needs, which really are very minimal, in harmony with the natural course of things. And practice total mothering with our sisters now. Every woman likes to be cared for with gentleness sometimes. Lastly, learn to mother your self, and be kind to our great mother, the planet Earth. This is the key to being in harmony with the mothering flow.

"Be not afraid to touch, naked body to naked body, to nurse often and orgasmically, to express your feelings as purely as your baby will . . . " - from Prenatal Yoga & Natural Birth

*A murmur is a heartbeating out of synch.

1. Hanrat Izrat Khan

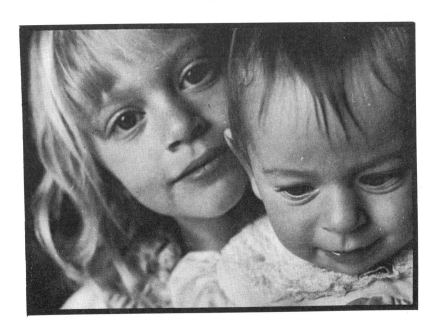

Placenta Recipes & Other Rituals

More than one woman has said that the reverie of our blood, for example, is a ridiculous over-reactions to many experiences of menstrual oppression. I agree. Yet, I *enjoy* the celebration! It is in this spirit that I offer some "Placenta Recipes", for your laudable information and edification.

The placenta is an organ surprising all members of the birthing family. It is also called the "afterbirth" and is never anti-climatic. It is beautiful to see - the colors red and blue are psychedelic! My fascination is shared by many native American women, and some believed that the way you relate with one's placenta affected future fertility.

I would guess that the majority of newly delivered women might not pay much heed to their placentas, especially *after* it passed from the body. But an ever-growing group of beings devoted to awareness, are obeying very old rituals about placentas. The Salish women on the coast of British Columbia would bury her placenta with a scallop shell, thusly, giving her a few years rest in between pregnancies. The **Cherokee** father would walk over as many ridges with the placenta as years they desired to not conceive children. There he would bury it deep in the ground. A lot of my natural childbirth students, with no placenta recipe to follow, so to speak, spontaneously decide to bury theirs. It's a rich experience - we buried one deep in the center of a circular garden one summer. However, many others elect to eat their placentas, vegetarians alike, though less likely on the whole. On cooking: prepare the placenta any way you enjoy(ed) the organs of animals. Liver, or better yet, kidney recipes are good starters. Read a few in the natural foods cookbooks and then forget them. When you first encounter the meat, remember to pause - placenta can be sacred food, if you let the meat tell you how to prepare it for the fire. (Raw is possible always - it's up to you.) The Paiute Indians thought that the woman might become barren if her placenta were eaten by an animal (or buried upside down to boot!) Were contraception this easy. . .

Chew slowly, till the placenta becomes a liquid, ambrosia. Placenta is a rare privilege for most of us.

July 1, 1977

Dear Jeannine,

This is about your inquiry concerning my letter to **Well Being.** You're welcome to use it. The recipe for the douche was an invention of my doctor, Jeffrey Anderson, M.D. of Mill Valley, Calif. It is a good one, he doesn't mind if you use it and doesn't care whether or not you mention his name but I think it would be nice.

It would make me very happy if you could let women know that a vaginitis which doesn't respond to treatment could be caused by hypoglycemia (or diabetes). Perhaps you could save others from suffering needlessly as I did. If you think it appropriate, I wish you would suggest a book **Hypoglycemia: A Better Approach** by Paavo Airola for anyone who suspects she may have this problem. Traditional medicine treats this condition with a diet high in animal protein but this can lead to protein toxicity because the human liver is not designed to handle so much meat. People who use this method feel better for a few months and then go downhill again. The best way to treat hypoglycemia is with a vegetarian diet. Dr. Airola explains this and why in his book. Since the "itch" is sometimes related to this syndrome it may be a good idea to include the information. You needn't use my name unless you think it important to getting the idea across.

I'd love to have a copy of your pamphlet when it is published. If you could send one copy for me and one for my doctor it would be appreciated.

Sincerely,

Laura

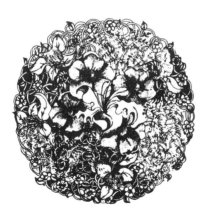

Appendix on the Hypothalmus and Some Hormones

I've resisted detailing the hormonal cycle as reflective of the menstrual cycle with its familiar curves on graph paper. To be honest, I wouldn't know where to start plotting a cyclical experience onto a straight line. This was some of the motivation behind the creation of the Natural Birth Control Mandala - to provide a journal more in keeping with the experience of **cyclical** fertility. When I want to explain the menstrual cycle and the relationship between hormones, feelings and herbs, the beginning always eludes me. Just where does the menstrual cycle begin?

.For uniformity's sake, writers and physiologists have chosen the first day of bleeding as "day one". Whether the intricate feedback system as manifested in the endocrine glands actually **start** with bleeding is unlikely. I've equally been fascinated with the consistent over-looking of the role of the hypothalamus. Pituitaries, for sure are being acknowledged in most popular courses on the hormonal cycle - but where is their friend and co-worker, the hypothalamus? We know that the hypothalamus is part of the limbic system. This is the area of the brain that is beneath the cortical, or "thinking" covering of the brain. The only sense that comes directly into the limbic system is smell. All the rest are mediated by our conceptions, our cortical processes. The sense of smell therefore, is called a more primitive part of our brains. Now what does this have to do with the menstrual/hormonal cycle in women? Firstly, it's been reported that women who are intimate, i.e. share the same household or retain a psychic connection with one another though they don't actually live together, oftentimes menstruate and ovulate together. Theorists have suggested that this is due to **pheronomes** - very tiny substances that females emit during phases of their fertility cycles and that are sensed by our sense of smell. A female moth, for example, may emit **one molecule** of this pheronome and attract to her millions of male moths when she is fertile. I have observed upon numerous occasions, how smelling an oxytocic herb (one that stimulates contractions in my womb) can set the familiar, rhythmic, internal massage of my uterus going.

Have you ever had the experience of walking into a room, from the rear door, to have every male head turn around to look at you, even though no one had seen your entrance? You might have been ovulating and emitting through the pheronomes signals to men that you are fertile. They pick up the message subliminally, i.e. without thinking about it first.

My hunch is that the hypothalamus is at the "beginning" of the menstrual cycle. In other words, the hypothalamus, concerned with such important functions as keeping an even temperature in our bodies (making **mammals** possible on this planet) is also very important in cyclical fertility. The hypothalamus is sometimes called the "seat of the emotions". Excited, it stimulates the desire apparatus in women —hunger, thirst, security, new experience - and the desire for sex. The desire for sex, pre-conditioned or before our sex-obsessed culture teaches us our "needs", comes part and parcel with the female's cyclical ability to reproduce. Now when I say sex, I mean intercourse here - semen into vagina - not the desire necessarily to be loved, valued, and touched. This explains, very simply, how women who are worried about the possibility of being pregnant can forestall their bleedings. The pituitary, the "master" gland for sexuality, lies in close enough proximity to the hypothalamus to be influenced by our desires. This is why when counselling women about abortions, getting pregnant, etc., my focus is listening to **all of the woman's desires** in the matter. I believe that a woman can desire a baby into being by not being clear about her very deepest programming - even if she is saying that she doesn't want to become a mother. Of course all babies come as an invitation from the mother and father during the act of intercourse - but what about rapes, parthenogenesis, and my lesbian friends who use contraceptives during their fertile times because they believe that their love is so creatively powerful that they could get pregnant, without any sperm? This is the hypothalamus talking here, in part. Surely our beliefs about where babies really do come from affects how we perceive the process. Currently our model is shifting from a patriarchal one (the quickest and strongest sperm gets to the egg first; survival of the fittest) to one of androdgyny (many sperms are needed to cooperatively dissolve the barrier to the egg). Yet beneath the beliefs are the desires, and the hypothalamus is sensitive to that.

*The hypothalamus is also sensitive to the onset of changes in the Earth's magnetic field (1) and the effects of solar activities. Other esoteric anatomists cite effects of the planets, **scientific astrology**, to which the hypothalamus responds. This is the connection between astrological birth control or the cosmically fertile time of each woman's month (2). Also, this "endocrine gland" is extremely responsive to changes in the blood supply from such disciplines as meditation and yoga practices. This is an explanation of how women who have a daily sadhana often become quite "regular", less emotionally "imbalanced", and able to produce "psychic miscarriages" by a concentrated meditation on the fetus and the imprinting of their desire for the baby to leave. I've included just one of many accounts of this process as a way of documentation of this extraordinary phenomenon.*

*I came across a remarkable sentence in **Esoteric Anatomy** by Dr. Douglas Baker. "The hypothalamus is extremely sensitive to the hormones appropriate to its sex. ...His **sexual continence adds to his blood circulation hormones of the opposite sex...** In women, there are newly won qualities associated with or permitted by male hormones like assertiveness, initiative, etc... It is not the hormones which give these qualities, rather they allow them to manifest more openly in the personality... science has shown that sexual excitation depends more on the brain than on the sexual organs (**and their hormones**)." Emphasis mine. This is the first feminist theory for continence that I've yet to read. He goes on to suggest, "Control of the hypothalamus lies in the reconversion of desire into will. We should never forget that desire sprang from will." This is keeping with the statements of my yoga teacher, Baba Hari Dass, that the world, as we see it, is nothing but our own desires.*

"True meditation implies control of the hypothalamus and all its techniques are calculated to bring about control, especially of sympathetic mechanisms and the gateway to them - which is the hypothalamus." (3)

*With some practice, I found after the birthing of my second babies that I could consciously control the "let-down" reflex of nursing. If I desired not to let down a copious flow of milk, I could concentrate on the middle of my forehead and with focused breathing to my pituitary/hypothalamus, curb the flow as long as I wanted. This was handy when my babies were newborns and the let-down of much milk would resemble more Niagara Falls than a quiet, simple feeding. "They" say that the let-down reflex in nursing is a conditioned one, implying cortical function as it is also culturally contingent - yet I've also read that it is an involuntary function in mammals. The hypothalamus is the meeting place of these two schools of thought. I have seen again and again in my practice that **energy follows thought**. If I think, concentrate with conscious breathing, on beginning my menstruation, I often will. How are the hormones implicated in all of this?*

*The two major female hormones are estrogen and progesterone. Not much is known about either. So I researched in the best laboratory/library of knowledge there is - my intuitive Self. For several years, I've been paying attention to the effects these hormones have on me during the various phases of fertility. It is true - progesterone gets me very high - i.e. perceptually I am functioning optimally. I feel progesterone coursing through my being during the lutein phase of my menstrual cycle and during the whole of pregnancy, especially towards the latter months. During the lutein phase, right after ovulation when the grafian follicle (the nest of the eggs) becomes the "yellow body", or corpus luteum, progesterone feels like the experience of falling in love. Rushes of excitement, openess to new ways of being in the world, and tremendous **gusto** for living. My senses are more keen - smells are even more powerful on my feelings and memories, touching, seeing, hearing, and tasting all are fuller. This mimics, in part, the experience of pregnancy, with the addition of emotional lability or the ability to feel a wide range of emotions in short spaces of time. As the corpus lutein cranks out progesterone from the ovaries, the possibility of becoming pregnant is with me. Here it is - the opportunity through my desires, to contain a baby. All women who desire to remain childless, might channel some of this creative energy into growing other things - like houseplants, for example. It seems important to move this (pro)creative energy through in action, by doing. Plant seeds in your garden - birth a poem or painting - mother someone you love - and fall in love with the Goddess, your Self. My hunch is that women get pregnant over and over again to keep getting this full rush of progesterone, to wallow in it, so to speak. It is difficult to let this hormonic feeling go, wind on down into a menstruation. But it is also part of the cycle - the life/death one and as we grow and expand to **our** magnificent potential, inclusive within this potential is the one for dying.*

Now estrogen is another story. Strutting is the single word I have for the feeling of estrogen. When estrogen peaks, leading up to the "fall" of ovulation, I begin to strut my "stuff". Men are now more important to me. My dreams have greater sexual content with them and all in all, I'm just more friendly. My ovaries feel as though they are smiling when producing lots of estrogen. Now hormones are simple secretions from an endocrine gland which act on a distant organ to alter its functions (or growth) and what makes an endocine gland different than other glands (like sweat glands) is the fact that it secretes hormones **directly** into the bloodstream. Estrogen goes directly into my blood - I feel "hot-blooded" at this time. Meditation is more difficult. The Follicle Stimulating Hormone, or FSH, secreted by the pituitary, is often picked as the beginning of the menstrual hormonal cycle - but don't forget that the hypothalamus sits directly over the pituitary. Occult teachers of anatomy refer to the innervation of the endocrine glands through the Vagus Nerve so that the parasympathetic system reaches hormonal functioning.[4] The Lutenizing Hormone, or LH takes a surge, which also isn't very well understood. You can begin to see how presumptuous it is on our part to take a synthetic hormone, or even plant hormone in great quantities and for prolonged periods, without knowing just what it is that we are doing to this intricate and somewhat mysterious process. We intuit that meditation on the Ajna chakra is helpful in regaining a sense of balance in our hormonal odyssey, and that much of the feedback control of the pituitary is monitored through the hypothalamus. The importance of the hypothalamus, and our integration of the hormonal experiences, will be ascertained in the next fifty years. Paying attention to this can only expand our awareness and further our evolution. D. Baker writes that the origin of the hypothalamus is linked with Atlantis. The evolution of this pivotal endocrine gland, I believe, is linked with bringing the experience of heaven here on Earth.

(1)   Baker, Douglas Dr. **Esoteric Anatomy** pg. 18

(2)   Jonas, Eugene **Astrological Birth Control**; also, **The Scientific Basis of Astrology** by Michel De Gauquelin

(3)   IBID Baker pgs. 18-28

(4)   IBID pg. 166

On Circumcision

Circumcision is painful. It is unnecessary. For mothers-to-be considering this "operation" ex bris or not, imagine having your own clitoris circumcised. This does actually happen in other cultures in the world - part of the human experience.

*And, one doesn't need to be circumcised to get into heaven. Heaven is right **Here and Now** if we but stop this hurting of one another and enjoy our bodies as the temples they are. And, it's been reported that uncircumcised men make better lovers. I've seen the "operation" - and say that anyone with feelings of respect for the life-force would not commit this torture. If the value be for initiation in some masculinely unfathomable way, then let it occur at the age of "reason" for little boys becoming men, with ritual and meaning. It seems devoid of much meaning to slice a newborn's penis, for aesthetics, for religions, or out of fear. Be quite clear of your own motivations for circumcision. There has been enough information published on this subject proving that it is actually a detriment to health rather than the practice of preventive medicine.*

I wish every parent who orders a circumcision for their son would watch one first. What feeds this phenomenon? My work in teaching yoga to pregnant women (so as to help them detach from the drama of the crisis; and not create a painful birthing), is aimed partly with this search in mind. What would cause a woman, fresh from the passion of birth, to allow her son's flesh being cut. Perhaps if she had been cut herself? C-sectioned, belly cut denying her the experience of the emergence by her own power - episiotomized, perineum sliced to enlarge the birth opening, numbing her the ecstasy of wearing the crown - pain, the mother's own pain in labor and birth turned back against the men, the baby boys, through circumcision.

Yet how do natural, gentle people delivering their babies with a minimum of violence, perform circumcision?

There is a strong tendency to conform among the birthing community. Whatever the popular myth, most new families will then act out wholeheartedly. The current myths are to experience during birthing, multiple orgasms and see God. And in some families, the present myth is to circumcise little boy's penises. I know a young couple whose relatives would come to visit from the East coast only if a son was born - and circumcised. A daughter would've warranted letters of congratulations only. She is not as exciting as a bris - the holy ripping off ceremony of Jewish boy babies in the name of God, our Father. Birthing, is something we can do privately in our homes but we must confront others whenever we change diapers. I would like to encourage parents of sons to confront, rather than continue to follow an old and violent tradition. We have found that our parents, our children's grandparents, still love us all - even without circumcising or delivering our babies in hospitals, or using formulas in bottles. As following anyone else's formula or program in birthing (like the expectation to have multiple orgasms and/or see God) is setting oneself up for disappointment, so is continuing to do violence to helpless babies via circumcision.

This is as heavy a statement against this practice as I can make.

Being Fertile

"I taste blood",
My lover says,
Ah! My first bleeding
Since the babies were born--
"I'm a 'woman' again!"
I sigh, satisfied.

Being fertile, in many minds, is linked with the concept of being a 'woman'. When does a little girl become a woman? Surely not before her first menstruation. Surely not because she takes a husband. Hopefully way before the birthing of a first baby, and before her first suckling of her child. A little girl is becoming a woman with each confrontation of her body as sexual -- and it is the blood which lends the "woe" to being a woman. As long as she is pre-puberty, sexuality in her experience does not consider the possibility of fertility. It is only with the bleeding that making love may come to mean in her body/mind the same as making babies. Some girls never do realize this connection -- **making love is making babies**, even as a remote possibility for themselves. I suppose that once we become "crones", as Ursula LeGuin tells us about the transformation (at 54 yrs.) of menopause (oftentimes coinciding with Saturn's second return to its natal position), the question is moot. But at the moment, when I am cyclically fertile, being aware of how I define myself as a woman and which experiences I allow of the multiple joys of female sexuality, seems very important. I am twenty-eight now and considering the possibility of never conceiving another baby. How will my woman-ness manifest without the intermittant "highs" of pregnancy, birth and breastfeeding? What else is there in life as **holy a process** as being a mother -- of sharing the **baby space**? When I live apart from other women and their children, a very interesting thing occurs -- I lose touch with this baby space -- becoming more irritable around **needing** little ones when by chance we do meet. Little human beings emphatically invite me into a here/now consciousness. I guess I am saying the children are my sadhana. Now this is fine, especially since we have agreed to a mother-child relationship already -- in other words, I've birthed and nursed three so far and see their needs for mothering lessening, just gradually, over the years. But that peak experience of birth! And the grounding of nursing ... these I feel attached to and love deeply. If my environment reflected psychic/sensual consciousness, as Shivalila describes, (1) the weaning from the "holy" process of mothering wouldn't be so traumatic for me. If sex with my lover was "tantric", like the Karezza(2) writers described, there would be no preferences to conceive or not, as a way of **getting it**. And as Berends(3) wrote: Trying to **get** pregnant, **give** birth, and **have** a baby isn't going to work-- the universe doesn't, in Truth, function this way. Surrender all this, and then you will **be a parent**. She didn't even write, "mother" -- **apparently**, identifying with the sexual in the process is also missing the point. So I must even surrender my attachment to this. Eventually I become more clear that it is not so much my attachment to **mothering** as it is my attachment to **opening my heart**. And all aspects of the here/now, as well as the cyclic/sexual dimension of consciousness, affords the opportunity to function as the Heart, in tune with the Sound, of love. Even with my tin ear, it is possible. And being a "woman", able to share the baby space which amplifies one's loving, it is imminent. And so-- women, sisters -- do not be afraid of the baby space. Do not turn off to the mother-within, the aspect of being which surrenders selfish desires in order to serve, and unconditionally love. Even those of us who are quite sure that we never want a baby (or ever again), continue to experience the baby space with all the babies coming in today. Baba Hari Das said that "children being born today need to be around people with open hearts." Mother those already here with us -- hang out with kids (I offer "mine"!) Often: it is a very powerful meditation. And this may be just enough reality to our fantasies of how nice it'd look to wear a baby on our hip -- when you've wiped their little behinds for the umpteenth time, all images fade into the now-ness of this service. And then we feel even clearer in our choice not to become pregnant, a highly recommended process for those of us practicing natural birth control. For it is oftentimes the mixed feelings about having babies, or not, that ends up with an "accidental" pregnancy. There are no invasions of babies -- the exception being rape (though some would argue even against this) -- nothing just happens *to* you -- like health, we create the whole movie. Babies come when there's an invitation via the act of intercourse. And I even know lesbian friends who say they feel like practicing birth control during their fertile phases also because **there's** so much creative energy. They're afraid that they could make a baby -- their love's that powerful. I do not rule out this possibility. If Mary could do it alone.[4]

Being clear that woman-ness is a consciousness that comes with the package, the one of being born female, and one that we are exploring deeply and that is always changing, brings great compassion. Compassion for **all** sisters, as each of us discovers just what being a woman means, and our responsibilities to this soul-making[5] process.

(1)   Shivalila Community, **Book of the Mother**, P.O. Box 1441, Bakersfield, CA. 93301.

(2)   Stockham, Alice B., **The Ethics of Marriage**, (available from Health Research, Box 70, Mokelumme, CA. 95245).

(3)   Berends, Polly Berrien, **Whole Parent, Whole Child**, Harper & Row, 1975.

(4)   Here we mention God, as the Father, for the first time. It is said by many wise men that God chooses when babies come to us. It is never our decision, in all Truth.

(5)   Hillman, James, **The Myth of Analysis**, Bollingen Books.
William Blake first coined this term.

Bump Stories

*After listening to hundreds of herstories concerning birth control and it's effect on our health, I'm developing a theory of iatrogenic practice by our birth control clinics, doctor's offices, public health agencies and alas, even feminist centers. To a surprising extent, we've maimed our bodies/psyches; and it is a large one, considering the frequency with which a woman's personal memory brought back deep feelings of pain, anger, and resentment. For the past several years, I've been introducing the conscious conception possibility to sisters and brothers through Healing Conferences and workshops. We begin a session with **clearing** - old stories about birth control practices are shared with the group. All too often, tears accompany several renditions. There are many women who suffer **bladder infections** with diaphragm usage, **ovarian cysts** with celibacy and IUD's, **traveling and perforating IUD's** with breastfeeding mothers, **madness** with the Pill, **warts** with froggy, sexuality-identification crises, **herpes** with sexual guilt, **vaginal infections** with over-indulgences, or conversely extreme horniness, and last, but not least, the **abortion dramas.***

*Abortions weigh heavy on many, many women's heads. Even the old 1967 Tijuana intrigues are sometimes haunting - and I discover quickly, that a woman cannot learn natural birth control, or conscious conception, if she is still back in Tijuana, one way or the other. So **abortion clearing** has become integral to teaching someone about their health, and responsibility to cyclical fertility. There are few women (who at least attend these California Healing, Yoga and/or Women's Conferences/Celebrations - of which my dear friend, Rosemary Gladstar, helped to establish) nowadays, who can say they haven't had an abortion. Taking the time to listen to someone's bump story, without judgment and with compassion, is a healing in itself. I've learned that the "symptoms" have much to say - so sometimes in workshops we give a voice to those venereal bumps. Instead of driving them away, right away, even by treating them topically with **sow thistle** or some other herbal wart remover, we **invite their message.** This way, every health crisis becomes an opportunity for learning.*

Dear Jeannine Parvati,

The sun is shining through autumn orange oak leaves, warming the cool morning. Little flashes of insect activity fly past my window and squirrels and jays call from the pines. The last of the pumpkins and tomatoes are in from the harvest. Winter comes.

And I finally sit here writing you. It's many months since you asked that I write down my abortion experiences, but some resistance has kept me from it.

After nine months, when I saw you, (at an herbal retreat), there was such a release, but it was not over and much was still held inside me. Now a year has passed since the abortion. The time of season has reminded me. A friend traveling from New Mexico to the farm to encounter abortion has reminded me. And those things that needed reliving have come and passed. So now I hope to grow and learn that no experience is ever over. Today feels like a good time to share with you and in doing continue to clear my thoughts.

When I got pregnant I was using a system that I myself called 'pressing my luck'. That was a loose rhythm that mostly involved knowing when I ovulated but not knowing why I knew exactly. It had been well tested for 1½ years with an irregular period. I was just beginning to tune into why I knew, the pangs, the changes in emotions, and mucous. I now realize I was on my peak fertility day but thought at the time three days before it and we were practicing Karezza, not coming, anyway. Or that was the plan. Mostly I remember unexplainably breaking into tears just afterward and having a feeling that I really blew it. Couldn't think of what to do so I prayed and put two vitamin (500 mg.) C tablets up my vagina in hopes of acidizing the environment too much for sperm. I was surprised that I was so freaked out, which freaked me out more. A week later I had a heavy infection that got herbal douched away. It felt like the vitamin C had not been too good.

I was working with a couple of naturopaths on my back problems and my late period fit in with it. I was drinking a quart of mugwort tea almost every day, was bitchy and thought I was crazy, but didn't realize I was pregnant until the day I left the southwest and the man I was living with to return to the herb farm. I drank pennyroyal tea but thinking back to all that mugwort felt it wasn't going to help. And pennyroyal is horrible to taste when you are pregnant. (The mugwort was too.)

Anyway, I was five weeks and that's too late for it. It was almost too late to have the simple suction abortion too. I never questioned that I shouldn't have a baby. I had prepared myself to face this long ago, but it was hard with all those hormones disagreeing with me.

I looked inside during meditation to find a soul linked with mine. To explain that it was the only thing that felt right to not have it and how very very sorry I was. But I never could find anything. It surprised me. I only had a feeling that the soul had known all along and was just playing out some karma for us both.

The abortion was very painful. I had an ovarian infection already and the area was sensitive. Also I didn't know I had a tipped uterus which made them have to do it twice.

And then it was over (I thought). I came home tired and empty. Took goldenseal, cayenne and cinnamon, lots of vitamin A & C, instead of the antibiotics and cleared up the infection and worked on clearing up my emotions.

But never did tell the father of that baby that I had been pregnant. My letters never expressed any of the fears or uncertainty or the resentment. I was a martyr and bore it alone. Mostly because I felt he was going through enough in his life and there could be no reason.

Nine months after I had conceived, or a few days before, I started crying - every day. And feeling more emotional waves than I had time to understand. And suddenly he was there. It was the first time I had seen him in eight months and he drove 500 miles to come and see me, but he wasn't sure why. Well, I wasn't going to break down and bother him with it after all this time, but I realized that I knew why he was there and **that making babies deals with men's psyches as much as women's.** hadn't copped to his role and he had come to claim it. So when we were talking and he said, "You should have a baby, it might be really wonderful for you. Your body wants one.", I cried and cried and could no longer pretend that it had not hurt me. When I told him, he said he too knew why he had come to see me, the universe tapped him on the shoulder.

It still needed time. I realize I shouldn't tell myself that I'm making too much out of it and must keep dealing with any feelings that occur. I'm very glad that I don't have a baby. I have had a succession of dreams involving babies that keep reminding me of a part of me that really would love one. (Or when I'm ovulating, 6 or 7 at least), I am very convinced that the ovulation method is the most reliable and certainly most tuned in type of birth control, if we do tune in. I am a fanatic in being careful to use it. (The universe seemed to tell me it has forgiven me long ago, now I just must forgive myself.)

I used BC pills for a year and an IUD for 3½ years and have had enough of them both. Just recently Linda had been fasting for a few days when she began bleeding. We decided that it was more elimination and she should drink beet juice but keep fasting. After two days, a piece of straight plastic came out of her uterus. She had her IUD out five months earlier.

When I called the health dept. about removing mine, she said "Some people can't put up with a little pain at first" and she knew someone who had one 2½ years! Then I told her how long mine had been in. She said, oh you must get it out and go on pills for awhile to give your uterus a rest. I couldn't help wondering if it is that hard on a uterus what was it doing in there.

I asked Hari Dass what was wrong with my back. He wrote, asking, if I had ever been pregnant, had unstable periods or been involved in problems in a relationship, and that the problem involved female organs. I see there is much work for me to do, to heal body and mind. To understand myself, especially in terms of being a woman.

This is from my journal:

October 1975

Reflections on an abortion
Sacramento's warmth feeling good.
The city buzzing around me somewhere   nowhere
Keeping up with so many changes in my body
Working off someone's karma, how many people's?
God, I want to find the soul who's living with me
    And none is there   nowhere
Maybe it's a token affair, a gift of some
    Bored one who saw I needed help
I do need help
Lead me so my path is clear
There is only one answer
    One head space
Filled with love and compassion
An' no room for you baby
You bulge my body
And spin my head

But I love you for coming, even though you knew
And I don't hate your father for coming
    Even though he knew
It is hard work but I'm keeping it clear
So I'm not going through this one
    Without learning my message
    Without keeping out those emotional clouds
And hear the lady saying why can't they give us pills to get pregnant
Hello my name is Amber
I look at the other women
I know they are pregnant, they know I am
    And I wonder if they look at me. I hope so
    Not wanting to be weird
Another office, 3 drahms of blood
    Does she know why I'm here?
    Can't see through the smile.
Seven nervous women smoking   talking
Alone I breathe   slowing down
Pride that it is so simple
    Until I find my breaths sucking in and out
    With that machine
Until the smiles disappear
    And my eyes close
And I hope I talked, enough
With this mush of blood
Holding a being almost not
Now surely not
And the lady is feeling sorry

Her hand pressed on mine
Not knowing the injection has left them
    Too numb to feel or more
She asks about my bracelet, if I made it,
I almost say, the baby's father made it
But remember it has just been sucked
    into that machine
But want to tell her that this all came
From something good. I loved him
And see he
Surely loved me and
Surely I'm not irresponsible - completely
And where is my head at -

Except must be crazy
  With pain
Then it's over. Oh God.
And I thank them eating their cookies
For I will pass out
By the time I get the raisins from my purse
And drinking tea
Wrapped in a blanket
Finally dropping pain pills
Trying not to ask why it was so hard
And glad it was so easy and over.

Wow, long letter! Hope this is of interest. I just started writing and all these pages appeared. I feel like thanking you for listening. It sounds like your center is growing. There is so much goodness in what you are doing. May God guide you, surround you with love, dear sister.

If you ever want to visit, please do, the Sierras and our farm welcomes you. And if you would like us to distribute your new book, I know without seeing it, we would like to.

In love,
Amber

Dear Jeannine,

The sun throws long shadows from its southern curve. Seasons changing. I follow the cycles in a perfection just beyond understanding.

Time of dying, casting off leaves and those sheaths that cover our **souls.**

The promise of rebirth still a seed.

Wrote the last letter spacy on fasting, releasing much, not thinking of it printed. So I responded with joy to share and fear also thinking of you using it - and my name. The "New Age" folk grow increasingly negative toward abortion with the whole macrobiotic/fruitarian/yogic/christain trips to back them. And feeding, reviving a little emotional fear of having karmically blown it. Ah, to be able to be clear enough within myself to not take on other's blame, for I am thankful to have had an abortion and feel strongly that each act must be not compared or judged, but taken within itself. It is each woman's decision to know if she can welcome and provide for that child. Hopefully, we will all realize that decision can be made at conception and that we are not enslaved by our cycles. . .

So all this head tripping to simply say, sure use my own name. And not my last name, since I rarely use it but my parents do and it would be unfair to their Catholic heaviness.

Thanks for sharing your experience with me, it touched me. I recently have becomed disillusioned by the great number of people I am encountering who are pregnant from natural birth control. Many of them admittingly made love when ovulating, as I did, others miscalculated they think (one using a diaphram when ovulating).

But I keep sharing my experiences and turning women on to the beauty of release from all those body infringing IUD, pills things. It is so exciting for us all, I want to believe in it. I am a fanatic, abstaining a week before and after ovulating (which dozens of reactions pinpoint its happening). But for many women this is too long to ask. I just feel using a diaphram is pushing it to the test when you are ovulating. My doubts are there about astrological fertility times although I observe them. When it occurs within a few days of my ovulation the stringy mucous extends their period. Otherwise I have no reactions and temperature at all, just nothing - to indicate being fertile.

More tuning in, more to explore! The universe unfolds in its own time.

May it shower blessing upon you and all our family.

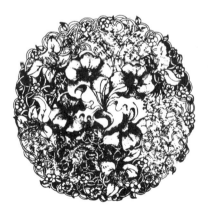

Namaste,
Amber

Some Thoughts & Feelings on Abortion
(OR You've Come a Long Way, Baby)
OR "You're Not a Baby and You Haven't Come Very Far at All"-Runes
by Tami Slayton Glenn & Jeannine O'Brien Medvin

"There is no 'correct line' on our bodies. There is no way to determine our 'real needs', our 'real' strengths and liabilities, in a sexist society - any more than there is a way to understand what 'female nature' may really be. How can we 'know ourselves' when the only images we have of ourselves are images cast by an oppressive society?"[1] from **Complaints & Disorders, The Sexual Politics of Sickness** *by Barbara Ehrenreich &* **Deirdre English**.

"Focus on how you **feel** *rather than how you look."[2] from* **Prenatal Yoga & Natural Birth** *by Jeannine O'Brien Medvin*

As Natural Birth Control educators, feminist health consultants and mothers of three a piece, the question of abortion is becoming part of our inner processes and dialogue.

Our counseling with women who have had abortions or who are contemplating one (or more) is prompting us to form a few thoughts and bring up a few feelings about the total abortion experience. We are becoming clear that abortion is not a simple physical process that is over and done with when the machine is turned off. Abortion is a metaphor for many of us on levels more than physical - aborted relationships, turning off to love, etc. The following thoughts & feelings are shared with the hope that a woman's experience may be enriched and enhanced through increased awareness of oneself.

First of all, it is our feeling that a woman who enters an abortion unclear about her decision and unaccepting of her choice will in some way manifest this conflict later in her life. Here **life** *as opposed to living, is a game of karma - the hindu precept of cause and effect. Our counseling suggests this in the following ways 1) chronic and unexplainable reproductive disorders such as pain in the ovaries 2) inability to fully participate in a sexual experience 3) a tendency to withdraw from social contact and involvement 4) a pregnancy following soon after the abortion that may demand a second enactment of the first decision thusly strengthening that samskara, or impression upon the soul. Some women have been able to make clear connections between their discomforts and their abortion experiences and others have not. We are suggesting that as women oppressed, we often continue to punish ourselves unconsciously, particularly via our "reproductive organs" and within our sexual relationships also, for our decisions unclear and misunderstood.*

1) Glass Mountain Pamphlet No. 2/ The Feminist Press 1973
   Box 334
   Old Westbury, New York 11568

2) Freestone Publishing Collective 1974
   PO Box 398-H
   Monroe, Utah 84754

For us, it is not a matter of whether or not to abort, but rather a matter of the awareness that brings a woman to that decision. Too often a woman does not give herself the space to explore all her feelings about this time in her life. Being pregnant "by accident" may very well be an intense statement to oneself and one best listened to with an open heart. The last woman we counseled became involved by sharing her fears and thoughts. By allowing herself that space she felt freer to make a choice unhampered by projections, images and fantasies, of how it might be, or how others might feel. This was one woman's experience and not necessarily suited for all. But significant because of the clarity she derived from allowing herself this process of sharing and exploring.

After reading a research questionnaire distributed from the Center for Reproductive and Sexual Health, New York's first legal abortion center, Bernard Nathanson, M.D., states "I read through questionnaires that had been filled out by patients, most of them young women, and what they seemed to express about their abortions was relief. No remorse, no regret, no sense of loss among 26,000 women. I found that a little alarming."

We too find this response disturbing. And our relationship to post-abortion women is indicating that there are feelings of loss and regret, that for various reasons are not being expressed. Our culture does not yet fully support or allow expression of deep feelings and through various images and ideas/myths keeps them down.

The months following the abortion, particularly the time at the end of the would-be gestation, can be significant. Women, sensitive to this time, have shared a feeling of giving birth to an aspect of themselves (a birth on another level) in their work, play or their relationships. By being aware of this process, they are able to support themselves and accept the changes they are

*experiencing. To have an abortion is not necessarily stopping the whole process, but saying no emphatically to one aspect of that process. There is a possibility that we may still be subjected to other levels of development initiated by the pregnancy. I once asked Baba Hari Das, our local realized being, if pregnancy on a subtle body level was possible and he replied with a smile of course and that one would then give birth to a subtle body baby. For **information's sake, he also knows that the soul inhabits** the body 22 days after conception.*

Our dreams can also be a rich tool for understanding our inner process. Dreams of babies visiting and communicating with us can be very illuminating. Our visions still include babies lurking in caverns and crypts - very early in my pregnancy I dreamed that I indeed was pregnant on all levels and a walk in an enchanted woods found me by a tree stump, a cradle for **another** baby. I didn't take to the idea, the reality of caring for two babies at once. So in a dream a voice softly said to start the adoption proceedings now to be well-prepared for twins. The rest is herstory - out of two conscious conceptions we have three children. Another aspect a woman can choose to explore is communication with the fetus.*

We have received this personal account from a sister first opened to the possibility of "psychic" abortion at a natural birth control workshop.

"One day it happened to us - we were pregnant and we hadn't intended to be. I felt ambivalent but leaned more towards himself and the child. Not a pleasant easy choice for either of us.

We acknowledged our responsibility in starting life. We had tried to prevent its happening, but it was there. A psychic told me it was a beautiful child and to think very hard before getting rid of it. Indeed, I could feel its power within me. I decided to include that tiny being in the decision of its future. "Little One", I prayed "surely you feel our dilemma. We don't want to destroy you, but we feel we can't welcome you joyfully at this time. Take whatever strength and energy you need from my body. May your stay within me be beautiful. If you feel you must be born then do what you feel you must. We are feeling that it would be best for you to leave soon. Please help us come to a decision."

Many times a day I would do visualizations of light coming into my womb. My conversations with the little one were endless. We had a good friendship and I shared with it all of my fears and dreams of motherhood. We grew immensely together.

After two weeks I had missed a second period and was getting anxious in spite of myself. Don was firm about not wanting a child. I now agreed with him, but the thought of an abortion sent cold chills up my spine.

One night I was lying in bed talking with the child. I thought I would tell it what an abortion was. I also wanted to run the scene through in my mind, in case I would discover that I now felt differently. I imagined being in a hospital. I imagined someone in white spreading my legs open. I imagined an instrument thrusting in and a tug. At that instant I felt a very sharp twinge of pain. I jumped. It was a sad and mystical moment. I didn't dare to breathe. Had it left? The next day my period started, deep red, full of clots. An incredible sense of loss filled me, and of relief. We thanked the being for leaving when it did. In those weeks we both came much closer to knowing what parenting will be for us.

I've asked myself why visualization worked for us when it didn't work for others. Who knows for sure? But I feel a primary reason was that we considered all three of us as important valid entities. Don and I didn't try to ignore a life we had helped engender, and we didn't try to will it out of existence by simply saying, "We'll get it removed." We considered the being in my womb as a personality with separate needs, desires and rights. We all three shared in the decision and we all three shared in the beauty of having been there together.

That spirit will always be our friend. Psychic abortions are possible for all of us."

We share this story as a means to illustrate a way of clearing the dynamics of a conception/abortion process and the reality of making it a positive, nurturing experience for all involved. It is through the awareness of the life energy that fills our womb and the respect we pay this life force and for our own bodies that can determine the quality of our experience. We feel it is possible to communicate with the fetus and very important to do so. Pregnancy is always a three way agreement between three equal beings - the mother, father and baby. Here is an example that underscores the importance of clear communication between the three players in a pregnancy drama. Another sister at the same healing retreat as the first we wrote of, told me that when she heard of the possibility of there being a birthing of sorts nine months after the conception of an aborted baby,   recollected that nine months after her abortion, the father of her fetus appeared unexpectedly at her doorstep. It seems the pregnancy was initiated just at the dying of their sexual relationship, when they often do - an attempt to unite through the physical and create a baby to further bond male and female together as householders - and her old man left without her ever telling him she was pregnant with their child. He traveled thousands of miles on an intuition and a deep desire to be with her nine months after that conception. She then told him about her abortion and his response was, "Now I know why I came." They, incidentally, re-established their love flow, without the bondage.

As science continues its relentless probing, we as the carrier of life will soon be faced with another decision. We quote Dr. Nathanson again - "Soon it will be practical to perform an abortion intended only to terminate the pregnancy, not to terminate the life of the fetus as well. The product of conception will be removed intact from the unwilling host - the womb of a woman who does not want it - and transferred to an artificial life support system that will let it continue to grow. The woman will surrender all legal rights to this child, and eventually the baby will become eligible for adoption. This may sound futuristic, but already we are salvaging babies at incredibly early stages of development. Some have been sustained outside the womb as nearly as 18 or 19 weeks. By 28 weeks, there are nearly 70% chance of survival. . . we will have a life-support apparatus that will allow us to sustain an embryo removed from the uterus at any stage of development."

Each new medical development that frees us from an unwanted situation also demands that we become more human, more caring for all involved. If given the choice to allow a fetus to develop in an artificial womb, (the final artifice), or die, it becomes implicit that we thoroughly explore our decisions. A midwife-friend of ours suggests yet another seed-thought about abortion. A woman who did not want to care for a baby decided to remain pregnant and give the baby to friends who shared the birthing and were willing to share the child with the biological mother when she wanted. Still emerging from the earth mother ideal, a bit fecund with romance, this seems like having your cake and eating it too. For we personally know the social reality of parenting is harsh at times - what nicer way to soften the incredible responsibilities than to share parenting with others deeply bonded to the baby, deeply loving the child, through the shared experience of birth. And besides, an adopted baby can learn to nurse from other women. Each pro-life statement we make with our bodies brings a sense of well-being. This is not to say that an abortion necessarily polarizes oneself or that it always is a statement pro-death. The letting go of an unwanted fetus may very well be a great celebration for your life. What matters here I suppose is best said as how you celebrate, the style.

*Is this the most loving thing you can do for yourself, your lover, your community? Our friend decided yes it was (unbeknownst to us - we didn't consciously know she was pregnant or that she had an abortion). The time she "had to go unconscious i.e. anesthesia and let someone else take the baby out as part of me still wanted to keep it", I was giving birth to **two** babies! The coincidence of her abortion and my bumper crop in babies has always struck us. Baba Hari Das in a personal letter wrote that when people imagine that they have control over conception they are in maya (in illusion) and those not having munity. This sounds right to me yet why me? I wonder, perhaps it was because one of us (the father) had emphatically said no to a pregnancy in an abortion with a previous lover, and this charge drew the double delight/duty of parenting twins. I check this out with my friend who just birthed two sons and she had had an abortion. A research topic for someone?*

This inner dialogue on abortion grows to a cacophany, blending in the multiplicity and merging full circle again/always. Our writing this for our community of beautiful women is a way to radically understand our own fertility and sexual realities. As householders, i.e. persons living/nesting and close to the soil*, the one desire we all share is to know ourselves as birthing/dying beings on all levels, in one breath, one heart.

* The sperm are reported to embed in the cervical mucus at the os of the uterus - in other words, lurk awaiting the ovulation to occur in the "crypts" which is a medical term too. Then the fertilization, and the birthing/dying danced by the egg and sperm a gratuitous miracle to feel.

*womb.

Dear Jeannine,

The first time I became pregnant, altho I was very pleased, my friends convinced me that to have a child outside of marriage would not work and was not right - and so, I received a series of injections of estrogen in an attempt to induce abortion. This was in 1967. There were no known side effects of estrogen therapy at the time (now it is associated with cancer in the child of the woman who received the hormone while pregnant).

The injections did not work - for which I was immensely grateful. This meant to me that God, as well I, knew this child was meant to be with me. Five years later this child had brought only joy and wisdom into my life, and so I could not but be happy when I conceived again, altho again, "out of wedlock". My condition was not excellent, however, after eating raw fruit and tomatoes frequently for three weeks, (after having eaten none for several years). This was the summer that I moved to Sonoma County. My body could no longer support a pregnancy. Those who understand yin and yang in relation to foods will realize from this that when a diet changes quickly from yin to yang, miscarriage can result. Most women are strong enough, however, that more than fruit and tomatoes would be required to cause an abortion. Ordinarily one would have to make oneself sick on sugar and other junk foods (extremely yin) in order to apply this principle.

1½ years later I conceived again. But this time I had just begun my first semester at nursing school and I was unwilling to drop out and have another child. However, I was also opposed to abortions - especially in the wake of having raised a child I loved so much whom I had tried to abort.

But I was very clear and unequivocal that this was not the right time. The intensity of my feeling directed me to lie down and go into a deep meditation state - such as I have rarely done before or since - for four hours. While lying on my bed that afternoon, I put my consciousness into my womb until I could look around inside and find the tiny fetus where it had implanted. It and I had a long talk. I explained how things were for me - that I wanted another child (this child), but not now. In the end, the baby agreed to leave. Sadly; matching my own feelings.

I got up (symbolically); drank my first and only cup of pennyroyal tea and went outside to run in the cool dark evening until I could run no more, crying out my grief to the stars. As I walked back into the house, I had a sensation of wetness - blood.

It is my conviction that anyone who really cares enough can do what I did. I have no special ability or training in meditation. Medical abortions foster irresponsibility and are violent to the organism. In fact, a woman is more likely to become pregnant again after such an abortion, for the fruits of her womanhood were ripped from her prematurely, and nature will attempt again what has just failed.

As for birth control, I have used a combination of ovulation method, astrological birth control, and a diaphragm on fertile days.

The only three times I have forgotten to take precautions or to check the calendar, I have become pregnant!

Carolyn

NOTE: Drinking large quantities of pennyroyal tea for several days is sometimes used as an abortant.

205

Menarche

The menarche are a passage surely not only into woman-ness but into being a lover as well. Menarche is an expression of woman's sexuality. Historically we've regarded **sex**, as **intercourse**, i.e. sexual relationships with men, not realizing that woman has five aspects to her sexuality[1] and not just one. Menstruation, pregnancy, childbirth, and nursing have the potential to be as satisfying acts of love and orgasmic as fucking. What I'm suggesting is that women's experiences of the menarche presently are more like suffering the visits of the Furies than an anointation of devotional nectar; surrender to the lunar flow that we've chosen, evidenced by being female bodies/consciousnesses, is being blocked by **our own images** and **cramps in breath.** This **passage, begun at puberty and lasting 'til our golden reign, at last a crone and relieved from going around the circleagain - this** passage called menstruation - sexualizes our beings and allows a magnificent opportunity to practice letting go. Menstruation-Weaning-Dying: the blood signaling that again this month the greatest attachment to oneself, a baby, wasn't conceived. The holds on our souls loosening with the bloody flow; a rebirth of sorts. A conception bonds you to those you love and a menstruation liberates you from life.

1. Newton, Niles **Maternal Emotions**
    Harper & Bros. 1965
    I don't believe Newton includ d the menopause or actual bleeding as sensuously pleasureable. And, suggested in the article "Trebly Sensuous Woman" th t there are other possibilities **inherent in female bodies** for sexual pleasure besides the obvious one (fucking). - Psychology Today

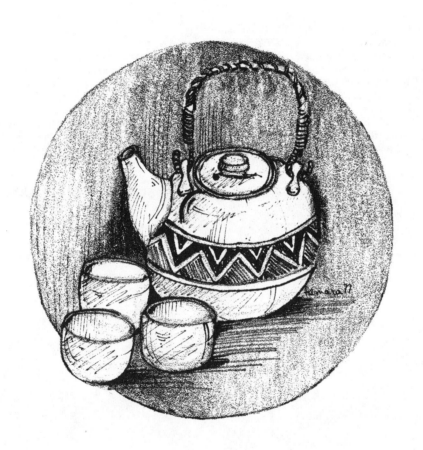

On Making A Book

As we three sat in the office of Book People (the distributors of HYGIEIA), about to sign the concretizing agreement, the image of how we put together our book came to mind. I saw us approaching the work of book-making in the same light as God making a planet.

This book has been gestated in my softest tissues of Self for many years. It began, as do all babies, as an idea. The original idea was that women are healers and have a particular style unique to our changeable, cyclical experiences of sexuality. The fertilizing agent, in retrospect I now understand, is my relationship with Tamara. We opened up the door to the imaginal world as a two-some and looked inside of these mysteries with all the enthusiasm and awe of any newlywed couple. What moved the enquiry at the beginning was the force of love. And what has borne out that initial idea is our evolving relationship. Unamuno said that only by personalizing an idea can we fall in love. By sharing those ideas most deeply attached to the core of my being with another person, the creative third was conceived--the book HYGIEIA.

The matrons for this pregnancy are our mothers. They provided us our grounding, the support, and the material means by which to share our work with you. At the most obvious level of involvement, they put up the loans to publish this book. On the more subtle levels, I felt corded and psychically nourished by my relationship with my Mom, Vicki, whose own example of strength inspires me still. It was our decision to have a homebirth, so to speak, of our book/baby to allow maximum purity in our statements and non-interference from established, patriarchal influences. Publishing one's own book, unless very wealthy (which we most definitely are not) is a risky business. As is a homebirth. Yet the alternative, big-time publishing houses, and hospitals, more often than not ask for compromises we wouldn't be able to make. I am pretty sure that our mothers were willing to risk their life savings on this venture out of their trust in their daughters more than their complete agreement with the content of our ideas. The generations may not need to see eye to eye--yet our levels of insight and how we view one another is from vantages of deep respect, honesty, and of course, motherlove.

Being a writer, which is a solitary form of self-expression, has self-pollinating, almost ingrown qualities, inherent in the process. By collectivizing my efforts and sharing the work, different creative possibilities came into awareness. The difference between masturbation and intercourse comes into mind. Which summons up the other seeming split in women's lives--that of being the wife to one's art, and the wife to a man--and the sometimes consequences of these marriages, the professional woman and the mother of children.

Through yoga, I am seeing how I adopt images, roles for the unfolding of my soul. One that is closest to me is the role of mother. With three young children, the time to adopt these other roles is very precious. So a good look into my attachment as the best mother for my children was called for at the onset of the writing of HYGIEIA. The muse coming was unavoidable--she necessitated that I allow other loving people into my children's lives in order to hear her fully. She said that I would be refreshed by my time spent with her and be able to more clearly value and care for my children by being apart from them occasionally. And so we formed a community, invited others to live with us and integrated our nuclear family into the newer model of physics. Yoga breaks down one's attachments to illusions–these years have shown me how complicated these false pictures are that mothers have carried about sacrifice. Sacrifice of their relationship to all the other Gods and Goddesses for the one of being the Great Mother. We are all the Great Mother, and those of us who literalize this by having children run the risk of forgetting that we are indeed more than this too.

And so I mother Tamara and she mothers me. This feels great too. Our baby is going through the last stage of labor now, called the transition. As in any process involving our souls, we have no clear picture of the who this baby/book will become over the years. We do know that what issues forth from us will have a life of its own, and perhaps, with the help of you, one day may turn around again and support us in our old age. What we ask of you as reader, is to give us directly your responses to the matter in this book, your feedback to our ideas, by writing to us. We cannot answer all letters personally, but a self-addressed, stamped envelope enclosed in your letter may facilitate a reply. And point of fact in the book business world–when you buy books directly from us, through the Box 398-H, Monroe, Utah 84754 address, the author and artist make more money than when you buy HYGIEIA through a store. Please do both, though.

To bring about the birth of our book, which is only the end of one formative stage of life, and the beginning of another, I now let go the last vestiges of false modesty. I must turn around to see my original face--and who greets me in this search are those two who made __me__ possible, my mother and father, and those two who made Hygieia possible, Coronis and Apollo (Epione and Aesclepius). To these divine parents, I release my attachment to HYGIEIA. And I thank you, dear reader, for allowing me this privilege of being "author"–for without you there is no purpose for me. NAMASTE.

Jeannine Parvati

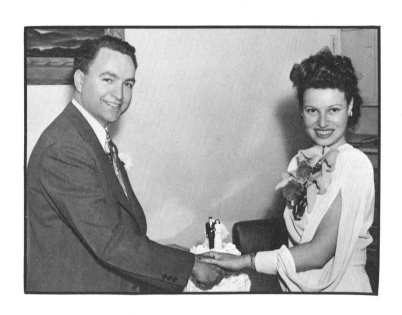

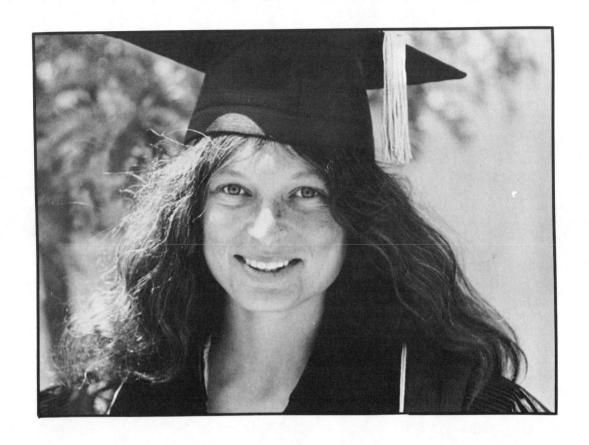

HYGIEIA: A WOMAN'S HERBAL

A creative project by

Jeannine Parvati

ABSTRACT

Purpose of this Study:

*To take the soul's point of view in an exploration of the feminine and healing was the task the Greek
Goddess Hygieia assigned to me. Her claim was that insighting into the mysteries of the female psyche
has been distorted through·our images of being sick and unhealthy. This has been abetted through our lost
connection with the natural world–the missing gnosis of woman as herbalist/healer.*

Procedure:

An alliance was formed between the world of plants and wounded women. The herbs, as psychic tool, were used to deepen an understanding about the healing process. Many old herbals and the present literature were found lacking of information for women. And so it was by application, with an eye to the mythic origins and reputations of any particular herb, that this connection with the feminine soul was established.

Findings:

Women have lost their faith in their ability to heal their own gynecological health crises and that this is a metaphor for the passionate struggle within the feminine psyche. Yet the relationship of being wounded and being healed is integral to any study of female psychology and that the information on Hygieia is heretofore elusive. It is a virgin field.

Conclusion(s):

Women seek out the experts when suffering to bring about an opening into soul-healing. By patronizing uncaring, cool gynecologists/obstetricians/psychiatrists, we are shamed into understanding what is at the root of the matter. Herbs are particularly powerful as a metaphor and grounds us in explorations of many aspects of feminine sexuality. This creative project may evoke the reader to re-vision the health of their own psyches. It is not my intention to medically prescribe--the herbs are presented for mythological and psychological value only.

PRODUCTION BY
TAMARA & QUILL

Just as I had no idea as to the immense concentration and energy it takes to pushout/let go of a newborn baby, neither had I the understanding of how hard it would be to finish this book. After months, years of conception, gestation bliss, the reality of hard labor was a bit difficult to accept.

The relationships initiated and sustained throughout the production of this book became the real creative process. A tiny backporch, transformed into a graphic arts studio, nourished an attitude of mutual commitment to what seemed a monumental task.

My relationship to Parvati, Quill, my mother, my ever patient husband and family, S.R.J.C. Women's Center and a world of women waiting to hear a new mythology concerning their health was my greatest source of inspiration. I am honored to be part of the revival of the "feminine in healing."

This book was blessed as a pregnant onion plant shot its blossom across my light table to observe the progress we made each day.

As an artist I continually struggled within the confines of 9" x 9", black and white. I found a space in myself that could be free yet restrained as I drew. For this, I lovingly dedicate the drawings in this book to Mr. Maurice Lapp, artist, teacher and wizard who continually shares with me the magic of drawing.

Tamara Slayton Glenn

erratic
ecstatic
process
pacing
erasing
ear racing
rising

Love fueled purpose
YELLOW sunporch Life
album of true dexterity —
venerable vessel
elemental vehicle

Thanks to Jack Robinson for the Mayan images & poem, for access to Sonoma State's herbarium, to Brian Elder for sources, to Mirian Cortez for humor, to my patient & generous friends & family, for ever loving balance. And to Phyllis Rausen for initiation & completion, much love. ♡♡♡

Quill

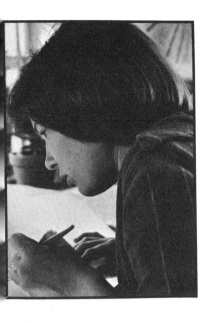

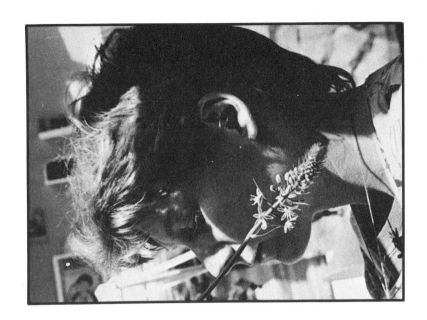

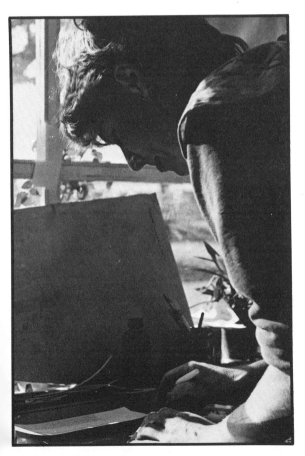

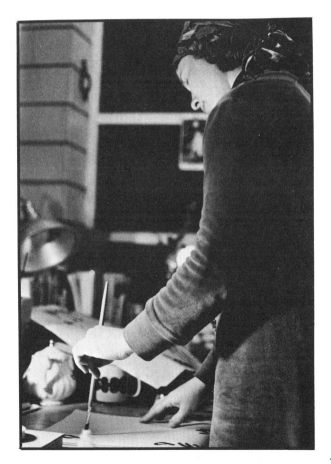

Thank you,
Art Warmoth, Ph.D.
Master's Thesis
advisor in Psychology.

He gave me the support
and space
to write this book.

To contact the author, write
HYGIEIA
P.O. Box 398-H
Monroe, Utah
84754

A Homemade Presentation
by The Center for Family Growth ©

and furthermore . . . . . .

 Actually it's best never to douche. Take sitz baths instead and by tightening and releasing pelvic floor, the herbal tea in the bath will soothe and cleanse the external genitalia and the outermost section of the vagina. By the time our daughters come of age, this "hygienic" practice of douching will be a relic of the past to the benefit of all.

 Bring the tea pot to the water and use no metal during any part of the preparation of herbal teas.

Tipped wombs are not causes of infertility - this condition is much more complicated than that. But as this positioning sometimes goes with sterility, doing something may illumine the root of the matter so you can see through to the meaning of a temporary experience of infertility.

 Acidolphilus taken as sitz bath alone is reported to be a superb vaginitus remedy by my women herbalist friends.

Parsley *Petroselium. Reported as an outrageous emmenagogue by Nan Koehler and Jeanne Rose. You take a fresh sprig and place it in your vagina. When I tried it, within a few hours my womb was contracting passionately.*

"The research findings as I have presented them **are very tentative and not at all proven**. In fact, it is my personal opinion that the research findings cannot be applied to the population as a whole, but only apply to a few individuals. In other words, marijuana, if taken daily and in potent amounts, **probably** prevents **some** women from getting pregnant, but its incorrect to say it affects the majority of women smokers that way." - Kay Weiss

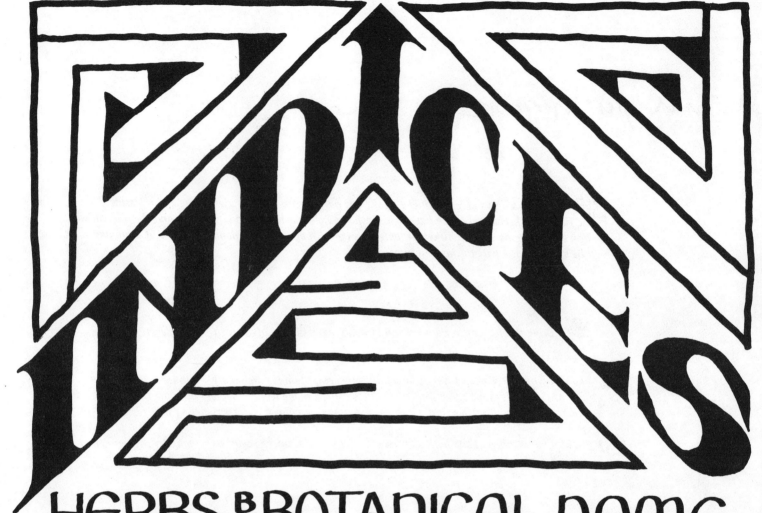

INDEXES

HERBS by BOTANICAL NAME

HERBS by COMMON NAME

AND A GENERAL INDEX FOR YOU

ON WRITING AN INDEX

In this index you will find many ways to identify with the material -- via ancestry (Greek, Hindu, Indian)*, myths (Hygieia, Aesclepius, Demeter), symptoms (vaginal infections, lovers, fear, etc.) and consciousness (dreams, intuition, images - to name a few examples). In some instances it's cross-indexed and categorized.

I especially enjoyed building the index, watching where each word would find her place next to another. For example "heart" was next to "Hari Dass Baba" for a long time - until "headache" came in between. Delightful metaphor for an aspect of my relationship as surrendering student of yoga.

And it also reads like poetry in some places... "Athena, attachment, avatar, Aztec..." or "understanding, underworld, uterus, vagina..." So on and so forth.

The categories are out of the main text, minus the Table of Contents, Glossary, and Bibliography. However, I did index the Appendices within the categories established in the chapters.

* by language - note no national or race references.

There are basically three indexes - Subject Index, Herb Index and an Index of the Latin names (botanical classification) of the herbs.

HERBS: LATIN NAMES

ACHILLEA MULLEFOLIUM L................Yarrow, Sneezewort

ALCHEMILLA VULGARIS R.................Lady's Mantle, Lion's Foot

ALFILERILLA Spp. ....Storksbill, Pinklets

ALLIUM ASCALONICUM ....Shallot

ALLIUM SATIVUM L.....................Garlic

ALLIUM SCHOENOPRASUM ....Chives

ALOE FRUTICOSA......................Aloe

ALTHEA OFFICINALIS M...................Marshmallow, Mortification Root

ALETRIS FARINOSA L....................False Unicorn Root, Star Wort, Colic Root, Ague Root, Star Grass

AMARANTHUS HYPOCHONDRIACUS ....Amaranth, Pilewort, Lovely Bleeding, Red Cockscomb

ANGELICA ATROPURPUREA L. ....Purplestem Angerlica, Masterwort,

APOCYNUM ANDROSAEMIFOLIUM ....L. Dogbane (Spreading), Milkweed

ARALIA RACEMOSA ....Spikenard, Indian Root, Spignet

ARCHANGELICA OFFICINALIS U. ....Angelica

ARCTIUM LAPPA C. ....Burdock

ARCTOSTAPHYLOS TOMENTOSA ....Manzanita

ARCTOSTAPHYLOS UVA-URSI ....Uva Ursi, Bearberry, Upland Cranberry

ARIAEMA TRIPHYLLUM ....Indian Turnip

ARISOLOCHIA CLEMATITIS ....Birthwort

AMORACIA ....Horse Radish

ARTEMISIA ABROTANUM ....Southerwood

ARTEMISIA ABSINTHIUM ....Wormwood, Old Woman

ARTEMISIA DRACUNCULU ....Tarragon

ARTEMISIA TRIDENTATA ....Sagebrush (Big)

ARTEMISIA VULGARIS ....Mugwort

ASARUM CANADENSE ....Wild Ginger

ASCLEPIAS HALLI ....Milkweed

ASCLEPIAS AYRIACA ....Milkweed

ASCLEPIAS TUBEROSA ....Pleurisy Root, Butterfly Weed

AVENA SATIVA G. ....Oat Straw

BAHIA DISECTA . . . . Desert Mallow
BAROSMA BETULINA . . . . Buchu
BERBERIS AQUIFOLIUM P. . . . . Rocky Mountain Grape Root, Wild Oregon Grape
BETONICA OFFINALIS L. . . . . Wood Betony, Betony
BORAGO OFFICINALIS . . . . Borage

CALENDULA OFFICINALIS . . . . Marigold
CANADENSE LINN. . . . . Erigeron, Canada Fleabane, Horseweed, Desert Trumpet,
Wild Buckwheat, Powa'wi
CANNIBUS SATIVA . . . . Marijuana, Grass, Weed, Dope, Maryjane
CAPSELLA BURSA PASTORIS . . . . Shepherds Purse, St. James Weed, Shepherds Heart
CAPSICUM ANNUM . . . . Cayenne
CARTHAMUS TINCTORIUS C. . . . . Safflower
CARUM CARVI . . . . Caraway
CASSIA ACUTIFOLIA L. . . . . Senna
CASTALIA ODORATA . . . . White Water-Lily
CASTILLEJA LINARIAEFOLIA . . . . Indian Paintbrush, Painted Cup, Pala' mansi or
Red Flower
CAULOPHYLLUM THALICTROIDES L. . . . . . . Blue Cohosh, Squaw Root
CENTAURA CYANIS C. . . . . Cornflower, Bachelor's Buttons
CHEIRANTHUS CHEIRI . . . . Wallflower
CHENOPODIUM AMBROSIODES . . . . Mexican Tea
CHEOROPHYLLUM SATIVUM . . . . Chervil
CHRYSANTHEMUM BALSAMITA . . . . Costmary
CICUTA MACULATA . . . . Spotted Cowbane
CIMIFUGA RACEMOSA . . . . Black Cohosh, Macrotys
CINNAMOMUN CAMPHORA . . . . Camphor
CINNAMOMUM ZEYLANICUM . . . . Cinnamon
CLAVICEPS PURPUREA . . . . Ergot
CNICUS BENEDICTUS . . . . Blessed Thistle, Holy Thistle, Thistle, Spotted
Thistle
CORALLORHIZA ODONTORHIZA N. . . . . Coral Root, Dragon's Claw, Chicken's Toes
CORIANDRUM SATIVUM . . . . Coriander
CORYDALIS . . . . Corydalis
CYPRIPEDIUM PUBESCENS W. . . . . Lady's Slipper

DAUCUS CAROTA L.	Wild Carrot
DELPHINIUM AJACIS	Larkspur
DELPHINIUM CONSALIDA	Larkspur
DICTAMAMUS ORIGANUM	Dittany of Crete
DIOSCOREA	Mexican Wild Yam
DIOSCOREA VILLOSA	Wild Yam, Colic Root, China Root, Devil's Bones
DROSERA ROTUNDIFLOIA D.	Sundew
ECHINACEA AUGUSTIFOLIA	Echinacea
ERIFONUM JAMES II	Antelope Sage
EUPATORIUM PURPUREUM	Queen of the Meadow
FOENICULUM OFFICINALE U.	Fennel
FOENICULUM VULGARE	Fennel
FRAGARIA VESCA	Strawberry
FRASERA SPECIOSA	Deer's Tongue
GAULTHERIA PROCUMBENS	Wintergreen
GENTIAN LUTEA	Gentian Root
GEUM RIVALE	Watrer Avens, Te Del Indio
GLECHOMA	Ivy Leaves
GLYCORRHIZA GLABRA L.	Licorice
GLYCYRRHIZA LEPIDOTA N.	Licorice Root, Wild
GOSSYPIUM HERBACEUM	Cotton Root
HAMAMELIS VIRGINICA	Witch Hazel
HEDEOMA PULEGIADIES	American Pennyroyal, Squaw Mint
HERACLEUM LANATUM	Masterwort, Madnep, Youthwort, Cow Parsnip
HIBISCUS SURRATTRUSIS	Hibiscus Flowers
HUMULUS LUPULUS U.	Hops
HYDRASTUS CANADENSIS	Goldenseal, Yellow Puccoon
HYPERICUM PERFORATUM	St. John's Wort
IPOMEOEA VIOLACEA L.	Morning Glory Seeds
INULA HELENIUM	Elecampane

IRIS VERSICOLOR	Blue Flag
IVA AXILLARIS	Poverty Weed (American)
JUGLANS REGIA	Walnut (Black)
JUNIPERUS COMMUNIS L.	Juniper, Common
JUNIPERUS VIRGINIANIA	Red Cedar (Eastern)
LAMIUM ALBUM	Nettle, White or Blind Nettle, Common Stinging Nettle
LAURUS NOBILIS	Laurel
LAVENDULA SPICA	Lavender
LAVENDULA VERA L.	Lavendar
LEONURUS CARDIACA L.	Motherwort
LIATRIS ODORATISSIMA	Deer's Tongue
LINUM ASTRALE	Yellow Flax
LITHOSPERMUM OFFICINALE B.	Gromwell
LITHOSPERMUM RUDERALE	Stoneseed
LOBELIA INFLATA	Lobelia
LOPHORPHORA WILLIAMS II	Peyote
LYSERGIC ACID DIETHYAMIDE	LSD, Acid
MALVA PARVIFLORA L.	Little Mallow
MARRUBIUM VULGARE	Hoarhound, White Horehound
MATRICARIA CHAMOMILLA	Chamomile, Camomile, German Chamomile
MATRICARIA PARTHENIUM C.	Feverfew
MELISSA OFFICINALIS L.	Balm, Lemon Balm, Beloved by Bees, Garden Balm
MNETHA PIPERIAT L.	Peppermint, Balm Mint, Piperita, Poleo
MENTHA PUELGIUM L.	Pennyroyal, Squaw Mint, European Pennyroyal
MENTHA SPICATA	Mint, Spearmint, Yerba Buena
MERCURIALIS ANNUA	Garden Mercury
MITCHELLA REPENS	Squawvine, Deerberry, Partridge Berry, Winter Clover
MONTANOA TOMENTOSA	Montanoa Tomentosa
MONOTROPA UNIFLORA	Fit Root, Ice Plant, Indian Pipe, Root Plant, Bird's Nest, Ova Ova, Corpse Plant, Convulsion Weed
MYRICA CERIFA	Bayberry, Myrtle, American Vegetable Wax
MYRISTICA FRAGRANS	Nutmeg
NASTURTIUM OFFICINALE C.	Water Cress, Scurvy Grass
NEPETA CATARIA L.	Catnip, Catmint

NYMPHAEA ALBAR	White Water Lily, White Pond Lily
OCIMUM BASILICUM	Basil, Sweet Basil
OCIMOM MINIMUM	Basil, Albica
ORCHIS CHIDACEAE	Orchis
ORCHIS MACULATA	Orchis
ORIGANUM MARJORAM	Marjoram, Joy of the Mountain
ORIGANUM VULGARE	Origanum, Wild Marjoram, Mountain Mint
OXALIS ACETOSELLA O.	Wood Sorrel
PANAX QUINQUEFOLIA L.	Ginseng, Panag, Osha, American Ginseng, Garantogen, Man Root, The Fountain of Youth Root, Flower of Life
PAPAVER SOMNIFERUM	Opium
PASSIFLORA INCARNATA L.	Passion Flower
PENSTEMON PALLIDUS	Palebeard Tongue
PETROSELINUM CRISPUM	Parsley
PEUCADENUM OSTRUTHIUM	Masterwort, Madnep, Youthwort, Cow Parsnip
PHARADENDRON FLAVESCENS	Mistletoe
PIMPINELLA Spp	Pimpernel Root
PINUS STROBUS	White Pine Bark
PIPER CUBEBA	Cubeb Berries, Tailed Pepper
PLANTAGO LANCEO L.	Plantain
PLANTAGO MAJOR	Plantain
PODOPHYLUM PELTATUM	Mandrake, Mandragora, Barass
POLYGALA AMARELLA	Milkwort
POLYGALA VULGARIS	Milkwort
POLYGONATUM MULTIFLORUM	Solomon's Seal
POLYGONUM BISTORTA	Bistort Root, Patience Dock, Dragonmouth, Snake Weed
POLYGONUM PUNCTATUM	Water Pepper
POLYPODIUM VULGARE	Lady Fern
PRUNUS PERSICA	Peach Leaves
PRUNUS SEROTINA E.	Black Western Chokecherry, Blackcherry
PRUNUS VIRGINIANA	Wild Cherry, Common Chokecherry

QUEROUS ALBA	White Oak Bark, Tanner's Bark
RHAMNUS FRANGULA	Buckthorn
RHODYMENIA	Dulse, Neptune's Girdle
RHUS GLABRUM	Smooth Upland Sumac, Smooth Sumac, Sumach Berries, Scarlet Sumach
ROSMARINUS OFFICINALIS L.	Rosemary Leaves
RUBUS IDAEUS R.	Raspberry Leaves
RUBUS STRINGOSUS	Red Raspberry
RUMEX CRISPUS	Yellow Dock, Sour Dock
RUMEX ACETOSA	Sorrel
RUMEX RISCUTATUS	Sorrel
RUTA GRAVEOLENS R.	Rue, Common Rue
SALIX ALBA	White Willow, Withy
SALIX NEGRA	Black Willow, Pussy Willow
SALSOLA KALI L.	Russian Thistle, Tumbling Thistle, Saltwort
SALVA OFFICINALIS	Sage
SABBUCUS NIGRA	Elder Flowers
SANICLE EUROPAEA	Sanicle
SANICLE MARIANDICA	Sanicle
SASSAFRA OFFICINALE	Sassafras
SATUREJA HORTENSIS	Summer Savory
SCABIOSA SUCCISA D.	Devil's Bit Scabious
SCROFULARIA AQUATICA	Figwort
SCUTELLARIA GALERICULATA L.	Blue Skullcap, Blue Scullcap, Mad Dog Weed
SCUTELLARIA LATERIFLORA	Skullcap, Scullcap
SENECIO AURUS L.	Ragwort
SERENOA REPENS	Saw Palmetto Berries, Pan Palm
SERENOA SERRULATA	Saw Palmetto Berries, Pan Palm
SMILACINA STELLATA	False Solomon's Seal
SMELACENA AMPLEXCAULIS N.	Solomonplume
SMILAX ARISTOLOCHIAEFOLIA	Sarsaparilla, Quay-Quill, Red Sarsaparilla, Jamaica Sarsaparilla
SMILAX OFFICINALIS	Sarsaparilla, Quay-Quill, Red Sarsaparilla, Jamaica Sarsaparilla
SOLANUM DULCAMARA	Bittersweet, Nightshade

SPHAERALCEA AMBIGUA	Wild Geranium, Storksbill, Alum Root
SPIRAEA TOMENTOSA L.	Hardhack, Whitecap, Silverweed
STILLINGIA SYLVATICA L.	Stillingia, Queen's Root
SYMPHYTUM OFFICINALIS	Comfrey, Knitbone, Suelda, Zuelda
TANACETUM VULGARE L.	Tansy, Golden Buttons
TARAXICUM DENS-LEONIS	Dandelion Root, Puff Ball, White Endive
TARAXICUM OFFICINALIS C.	Dandelion Root, Priest's Crown
TAUXUS BACCATA	Yew
TETRADYMIA CANESCENS INERMIS	Wuta' Kvala
THYMUS SERYPHYLLUM L.	Creeping Thyme, Mother of Thyme
THYMUS VULGARIS	Thyme
TRIFOLIUM PRATENSE L.	Red Clover
TRIGONELLA FOENUM GRACECUM	Fenugreek Seed
TRILLIUM PENDULUM	Beth Root, Birth Root, Milk-Ipecac, Lamb's Quarter, Jew's Harp Plant, 3 Leafed Nightshade
TROPOELUM MAJUS	Nasturtium
TURNERA APHRODISIACA	Damiana
TROPOELUM MAJUS	Nasturtium
TURNERA APHRODISIACA	Damiana
ULMUS FULVA	Slippery Elm Bark
URTICA DIOICA	Nettle
USTILAGO ZEAE	Corn Smut
VALERIANA OFFICINALIS	Valerian
VANILLA PLANIFOLIA	Vanilla
VERATRUM CALIFORNICUM E.	False Hellebore
VERBENA HASTATA	Verbena, Vervain, Wild Hyssop
VERBENA OFFICINALIS V.	Verbena, Vervain, Wild Hyssop
VIBURNUM OPULUS	Cramp Bark, American Sloe, Highbrush Cranberry
VIBURNUM PRUNIFOLIUM	Black Haw
VINCA Major & Minor APOCYNACEAE	Periwinkle
ZINGIBER OFFICINALIS	Ginger Root

HERBS : COMMON NAMES

GENERAL INDEX

NURSING   17, 32, 37, 40, 71, 77, 80, 93, 95, 97, 107, 108, 117, 121, 123, 124, 126, 172, 173, 185, 186, 190,
193, 203, 206 See Breastfeeding & Lactation
NUTMEG   23 (See Herb Index - Use sparingly - Rolling Thunder considers it poisonous.)
NUTRITION - NUTRIONISTS   11, 14, 32, 45, 89, 92, 95, 97 (mal), 107, 117, 122, 125, 127, 137, 138, 139,
142, 183

OBSTETRICS-OBSTETRICIAN v, 3, 39, 82, 110, 112, 115, 131, 212
OCCULT   85, 107, 191
ODYSSEUS   76
OJAS   11
OLYMPUS ix
ORGASM   11, 74, 81, 95, 141, 178, 186, 192
OVARY-OVARIAN   14, 24, 27, 34, 39, 56, 77, 89, 91, 102, 105, 120, 121, 125, 137, 138, 139, 190, 191,
195, 196, 201 By Symptom Disorders 89, Dysfunction 34, 77, Ailing 125, Cysts 39
Trouble 24, 102 By Herb: 24 Blue Cohosh, 27 Pennyroyal, 56 Blue Cohosh,
77 Saw Palmetto Berries, 102 Black Cohosh, 120 Bayberry, 121 Burdock, 125 Peach Leaves
OVULATION-TO OVULATE   11, 34, 37, 40, 57, 79, 81, 92, 95, 96, 97, 109, 123, 126, 133, 134, 138, 171,
172, 173, 174, 180, 189, 190, 191, 196, 197, 200, 205
OVUM   8, 65, 170 See Egg
OXALIC ACID   45
OXYTOCIN-OXYTOCIC   35, 107, 189

PAIN   iv, 5, 8, 14, 23, 24, 26, 27, 28, 29, 34, 42, 52, 57, 58, 61, 63, 74, 77, 90, 92, 95, 96, 99, 102, 103,
104, 105, 106, 115, 120, 121, 125, 127, 128, 129, 142, 185, 192, 195, 196, 197, 199, 201, 203
By Symptom: of Childbirth 23, relieves 24, of Menses & Afterbirth Pains 26, in Genitals & Hips
28, in Childbirth 58, Menses 77, Bladder Infection 90, Vaginitus 92, Yeast Infection 95, Lower Back 96,
Menses 99, 102 & in Birth 103, Menses 104, Griping 106, Painless Childbirth 115, in Childbirth 120,
121, in Uterus 122, Gas & Menses 125, in Childbirth 128, in Pregnancy 129, in Circumcision 192
By Herb: 23 Basil, 24 Catnip, 26 Little Hallow, Masterwort & Mexican Tea, 27 Common Rue
(caution in use during pregnancy), 28 Thyme, 58 Wild Ginger, 77 Wild Carrot, 96 Blue Cohosh,
99 Balm, 105 Ragwort, Thyme, 58 Wild Ginger, 77 Wild Carrot, 96 Blue Cohosh, 99 Balm,
105 Ragwort, 102 Coral Root & Cotton Root 103, 104 Motherwort, 105 Myrrh & Ragwort, 120
Black Western Chokecherry, 121 Buckwheat 125 Balm Mint, 127 Smooth Upland Sumac, 128 St. John's
Wort, Wild Cherry & Wild Ginger, 129 Wild Yam
PANACEA ix, 103
PARACELSUS   42

from our family to yours:

      Since writing this book, quite a few years ago now.........
I have become more deeply involved in lay midwifery and woman's self-health-care. Out of this involvement has come several other writing projects in progress.

      In order to share more of this information HygieiaCollege was formed, devoted to women healing women and will now be available as a complete correspondance course in midwifery and womancraft.

= Please write for more information. =

      With all this, PRENATAL YOGA continues to do well - the Goddess has been gracious - and I also want to thank YOU ALL for the wonderful support.

      Blessed Be,

          Jeannine

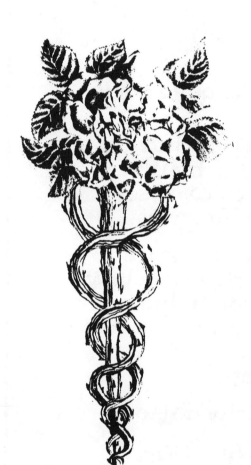

hygieia college

CORRESPONDENCE · COURSE

with · Jeannine Parvati Baker ·

●

Self paced home study in Womancraft and Lay Midwifery · Healing Birth Naturally at home and beyond · Ten Lessons to guide You to the Sources of Feminist Alchemy · Including in depth study of:

herbalism · sexuality · mythology · consciousconception · dreams politics · visions · lotus birth astrology · pressure points · touch tantric yoga · chants · sounds

Introduction to the maiutic process of education (in the manner of a mid-wife) with personal evaluative dialog as needed on each lesson.

●

$500 for all ten lessons or **$60** each lesson

SEND $50 FOR SAMPLE LESSON
#1 · THE INNERVIEW
P.O. BOX 398
MONROE · UTAH · 84754 · H

.... Blessed Be ....

FREESTONE INNERPRIZES

also known as the Center for Family Growth & The Alchemical Bakery

Books from Freestone include:

Conscious Conception

Conscious Conception is a multi-perspective view of the reproductive experience, a rich tapestry of personal sharings, natural methods of contraception, mythology, religion, the dream state and much more.

416 pp, 8½ x 11, paper, 3rd printing

Prenatal Yoga and Natural Birth

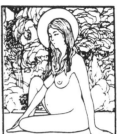

Hatha yoga exercises for pregnant women are an ideal way to prepare for childbirth. Jeannine Parvati, who is a practicing midwife, yoga teacher, feminist health counselor and mother of six children, has adapted the esoteric practices of yoga for pregnant women with no previous exposure to the exercises, breathing and meditation. The book is useful for the advanced student as well as the beginner. Clear directions and plenty of photos & illustrations.

96 pp, 8½ x 11, paper, 2nd edition 1986

These books can be ordered directly or through your favorite book or health food store. If you know our books & enjoy them, please ask your local stores & libraries to carry them. Thank you and blessed be.

relatives of Freestone Publishing Collective:

Freestone Innerprizes

Distribution of books, articles, recorded college courses on the general theme of feminist, healing, psychological, home birth & rebirth of parents & children.

Hermetic Astrology & Psychology

Astrology tapes & charts specializing in family and relationships, health counseling, myth and story are accented. Cassettes may be ordered by mail for your convenience.

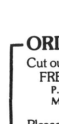

Hygieia College

Classes and workshops in Lay Midwifery, Gyn/Ecology, Healing Women, Holistic Health for Babies, Astrology, Dream Groups, Women's Magic, Herbalism, Natural Birth & (Trans) Parenting. NOW AVAILABLE AS A CORRESPONDANCE COURSE.

ORDER FORM

Cut out or send reasonable facsimile to:
FREESTONE INNERPRIZES
P. O. Box 398-H
Monroe, UT 84754

Please send me:
- ☐ Prenatal Yoga @ $10 + $2
- ☐ Hygieia @ $15 + $2.50
- ☐ Conscious Conception @ $20 + $3
- ☐ more info about Hygieia College -and correspondance course
- ☐ catalog of tapes, articles, & books ($2—refundable)
- ☐ more info on Hermetic Astrology & Psychology
- ☐ I would like to be on your mailing list and receive info periodically

NOTES